babygate

Acclaim for *Babygate*

"Any mother-to-be who buys *What to Expect When You're Expecting* should pick up a copy of *Babygate* to go with it. It offers indispensable advice to allow working parents to stay on the job and is a blueprint for change in the coming work–family revolution."

—Anne-Marie Slaughter, Princeton University professor and author of *Why Women Still Can't Have It All*

"A Better Balance, one of the outstanding defenders of parents' legal rights in the United States, has given us an indispensable guide with *Babygate*. No new parent should leave the hospital without it!"

—Ann Crittenden, Pulitzer Prize nominee and author of *The Price of Motherhood*

"If you're a working parent, you need *Babygate*—an invaluable and humane guide for expecting and new parents about their legal and economic rights in the American workplace. The information in its pages will provide answers to your most important questions and empower you to stand up for yourself and working families."

—Katrina vanden Heuvel, editor and publisher of *The Nation*

babygate

HOW TO SURVIVE PREGNANCY AND PARENTING IN THE WORKPLACE

DINA BAKST

PHOEBE TAUBMAN

ELIZABETH GEDMARK

THE FEMINIST PRESS
AT THE CITY UNIVERSITY OF NEW YORK
FEMINISTPRESS.ORG

Published in 2014 by the Feminist Press
at the City University of New York
The Graduate Center
365 Fifth Avenue, Suite 5406
New York, NY 10016

feministpress.org

First printing September 2014

Cover design by Jenifer Walter
Text design by Drew Stevens
Icon design by Suki Boynton

Library of Congress Cataloging-in-Publication Data
Bakst, Dina, author.
Babygate : how to survive pregnancy and parenting in the workplace / by Dina Bakst, Phoebe Taubman, and Elizabeth Gedmark.
pages cm
Includes state-by-state guide.
Includes bibliographical references.
ISBN 978-1-55861-861-9 (pbk.) — ISBN 978-1-55861-862-6 (ebook)
1. Mothers—Employment—Law and legislation—United States. 2. Pregnant women—Employment—Law and legislation—United States. 3. Working mothers—Legal status, laws, etc.—United States. 4. Parental leave—Law and legislation—United States. 5. Discrimination in employment—Law and legislation—United States. I. Taubman, Phoebe, author. II. Gedmark, Elizabeth, author. III. Title.
KF3467.B35 2014
650.1085'20973—dc23

2014020052

CONTENTS

FOREWORD

Cynthia Thomas Calvert and Joan C. Williams

As pioneers in the fight to eliminate family responsibilities discrimination, we hear a lot of stories from women who were successful at work until they became pregnant. We hear from women who announced their pregnancies and were soon reassigned to dead-end jobs, disciplined for made-up infractions, harassed, demoted, and terminated. We hear from women with young children who have been passed over for promotions, given unfairly negative performance evaluations, punished for things other employees are not, and pushed to the sidelines. These stories confirm what our research shows: the strongest form of sex discrimination in the workplace today is discrimination against women who are mothers or are pregnant.

We have come to the conclusion that employers may know that it is illegal to discriminate against women because they are women, but many do not know that it is illegal to discriminate against women because they are or soon will be mothers. We're working to change that, but in the meantime, women need to arm themselves with as much information about their legal rights as possible. *Babygate: How to Survive Pregnancy and Parenting in the Workplace* is an enormously useful tool to help women learn what protections they have under the law and how to address maternal wall discrimination with their employers. It provides essential information about federal and state laws in plain English, covering everything from pregnancy and nursing to parenthood and flextime. The legal discussion is complemented by practical tips and tools, ensuring that readers will know what to expect and will be prepared to meet challenges at work. The authors provide real-life examples of other women's experiences throughout, making this book inspirational as well as instructive.

The authors' goal, and ours, is to eliminate the legal obstacles and biases that hold women, particularly mothers and pregnant women, back from achieving full equality in the workplace. *Babygate* is an important contribution toward making this goal a reality. As women implement its lessons in the workplace, the experiences and attitudes of employees and employers will begin to change. Supervisors and colleagues will see that mothers who are treated fairly become loyal and committed, flexible schedules work and can benefit the company, and whole human beings with robust family lives are better and more productive workers. Men gain alongside the women, not only from having a more profitable employer but from being freed to have more well-rounded lives themselves.

Women are poised to break through the glass ceiling: we are 50 percent of the workforce, more than 50 percent of college graduates, and we earn more advanced degrees. That is what makes this book so timely and necessary. By pointing out ways around, over, and through the maternal wall, *Babygate* can help women survive at work while the wall is being torn down. And as more women get through the wall, the wall will come down faster.

PREFACE

Dina Bakst, Phoebe Taubman,
and Elizabeth Gedmark

As an expecting parent, you're likely to encounter a dizzying array of information and advice about how to incubate, birth, and raise a healthy child. What to expect from your body during your pregnancy? There's a book for that. Natural child-birth? Check. Sleep training? There's a method for everyone. But when problems crop up at work because of your pregnancy or parenthood, where do you turn?

Although women entering the workplace today start their careers better educated than their male peers and at near parity in wages, they fall behind when they become mothers (more than 80 percent of women in the United States have children by the time they're forty-four years old). Studies show pregnant women and mothers experience widespread wage and hiring discrimination and only a fraction have access to paid sick time and family leave to care for a new child. Simply put, pregnancy is a key trigger for inequality that endures across a woman's lifetime: motherhood is the biggest risk factor for poverty among women in old age. This is the shameful status quo in the United States in 2014.

In 2005, Dina Bakst cofounded A Better Balance (ABB): The Work and Family Legal Center with a group of fellow women's rights lawyers to tackle this problem. Together they wanted to strengthen legal protections for caregivers and to promote policies that allow all workers, particularly pregnant women and new mothers, to care for their families without risking their financial security. A Better Balance, where all the authors of this book work, is dedicated to promoting fairness in the workplace and has become a leader in the fight to expand paid leave for parents and caregivers, combat workplace discrimination based on pregnancy and family status, and increase access to flexible and predictable work schedules.

We are happy to report that we are making substantial headway on all of these fronts with incredible legislative victories. Over the past year, A Better Balance drafted Rhode Island's successful family leave insurance law—the third of its kind in the country—and helped advance the federal FAMILY Act, which proposes to fund paid family leave for all Americans. We recently shepherded new laws guaranteeing paid sick time to workers in Portland, Oregon; Jersey City and Newark, New Jersey; and in our own hometown of New York City. We secured groundbreaking legal rights for pregnant women in New York City, and advanced similar laws in New Jersey, Minnesota, and West Virginia, so workers can stay healthy and employed when they need a modest accommodation, including time off to safely recover from childbirth. And we supported San Francisco legislators as they passed one of the first workplace flexibility laws in the country. We also opened our A Better Balance Southern Office, based in Nashville, TN, to bring our successful model of advocacy and direct services where it is greatly needed. There is still so much work to be done, but we are excited about the momentum we see.

Although the core of our advocacy is focused on policy change, we have always been committed to educating the public and helping individuals understand their legal rights. *Legislation is only effective when workers know about their rights and feel confident using them when needed.* Unfortunately, confusion is widespread: for example, in one of our recent trainings in New York, not one participant was certain whether she had a legal right to pump breast milk at work. In fact, half the room thought it was acceptable for a boss to insist a nursing mother pump breast milk in a bathroom stall. It's no wonder: the internet is chock-full of misinformation, and too many workers, especially those in low-wage, inflexible jobs, cannot rely on the goodwill of their employers to make sure they're treated fairly.

In 2009, we launched a free legal clinic in New York for low-income workers who have problems at work related to their pregnancy and family responsibilities. Since then we've received hundreds of phone calls from men and women with questions about parental leave, pregnancy discrimination, sick time, flexible work, and dozens of other issues. We've counseled workers about how to speak with their bosses, where to apply for benefits, and how to protect themselves when they suspect discrimination. We convinced one of the largest employers in Brooklyn to change its policy to allow pregnant women who could still do their jobs with accommodations to continue working, and helped an expecting mother get back on her feet after she was forced out of work and into a homeless shelter. Some of the women we have counseled have joined our advocacy as well, harnessing their stories and their passion as agents for change.

We love this work, but as a small organization we have limited capacity to offer personal assistance to everyone in need. We wanted to extend our reach to a broader audience of people across the country who, like our callers, are confused about their rights or simply do not know how existing laws could help them stay on the job. Where is the book for this, we wondered? And thus, *Babygate* was born.

We wrote *Babygate* to provide a comprehensive resource for expecting and new parents about their workplace rights and to fill a gap in the canon of parenting literature. But we had another motive as well. While *Babygate* is a tool for self-help, individuals cannot, and should not, be expected to solve what is, fundamentally, a systemic problem of work–family incompatibility. Throughout this book we highlight how poorly the United States stacks up against other countries when it comes to supporting working families and how dramatically worker rights and protections vary by state: for example, pregnant and new mothers in New York are entitled to a maximum disability payment of $170/week if they cannot work while pregnant or recovering from childbirth, while mothers in California may receive up to $1,075/week and up to four months of job-protected leave. Our goal is to educate but also to inspire a bit of outrage. In fact, we chose the title *Babygate* to evoke the idea of a scandal. Why is the richest country in the world also one of only a handful without any guarantee of paid time off for new mothers? Why, in 2014, are we still fighting for the ability to stay home when we, or our children, are sick without risk of losing income or a job? Why do news stories about work and family consistently focus on women's choices, and not on the structures of outdated policies and social institutions that constrain those choices?

We believe that mothers, fathers, sons, daughters, and other family caregivers deserve better. Our economy is built on their invisible and free labor, whether it is the education and socialization of the next generation of workers or the comfort and care of the elderly. We all benefit from this resource, and yet, as a society, we take it for granted and do little to ensure its continued vigor. Our work at A Better Balance, and this book, is dedicated to changing that reality.

Blending work and parenthood is a constant challenge—we know; we've been there. Although there is no perfect solution, we hope *Babygate* can provide some answers. We hope the pages that follow will inform and empower you, giving you the confidence to stand up for yourself at work and the inspiration to stand up for working families everywhere.

babygate

INTRODUCTION

Are you pregnant or thinking about taking that step? Maybe your partner is pregnant, and you are trying to plan for the big changes that await you. Or perhaps you are eagerly anticipating a new baby through adoption. No matter how you got here, welcome!

You've probably been reading about what to expect from pregnancy and how to prepare for childbirth. Maybe you've even started thinking about the early days of parenthood and how to care for your new baby. We are here to help you learn about your legal rights as an expecting or new parent. Specifically, we want to help you plan how to integrate pregnancy and parenthood into your work life. How do you plan for maternity/parental leave? What are you entitled to? What do you do if you suspect workplace discrimination? What if you want to work part-time after your child is born?

Don't know the answers to these questions? You are not alone. We work on these issues every day and talk with plenty of people who don't understand their rights as working parents. Many more don't realize how limited their rights are in comparison to the rights of parents in other countries around the world. For example, we got a call to our hotline from a woman who was born in Denmark, where parent-friendly laws are the norm. Helena was now living in the United States and was pregnant with twins. She worked for a small company that didn't offer any paid maternity leave. Her boss wanted her to return to work two weeks after her babies were born, but Helena (understandably) wanted more time to recover from giving birth and to bond with her newborns. Helena couldn't get much information out of her employer, but she thought she was entitled to twelve weeks of unpaid leave under federal law. Unfortunately, because her employer was too small to be covered by the law, Helena had no guarantee of time off. When we broke this news to Helena, she was shocked. She couldn't believe that a country as rich as the United States, whose politicians profess their commitment to family values, could leave someone like her in the lurch—and at such a critical moment in her life.

Helena's situation is all too common in the United States, where parental leave, child care, and flexible work schedules have been left largely to employers and employees to work out on an individual basis. As we describe in more detail throughout this book, there are some federal laws to protect employees and lots of state laws too, but mostly employers still call the shots. And in a struggling economy many employers have cut back on what limited benefits they do provide to employees, making the situation that much worse for expecting and new parents.

On top of all this, bias against pregnant women and new mothers is still a serious problem in the United States, despite the fact that Congress outlawed discrimination based on pregnancy about thirty-five years ago. Apparently, many employers haven't gotten the memo. The Equal Employment Opportunity Commission (the federal agency that enforces the law) saw a steady increase in charges of pregnancy discrimination over the decade between

2000 and 2010: complaints jumped by 50 percent. And according to a recent MSNBC poll of over 7,000 people, more than 62 percent have personally seen or experienced workplace discrimination against pregnant women.[1] By that measure, pregnancy discrimination is the norm, not the exception, in today's workplaces. Given that women make up half of the workforce, and 80 percent of American women will become pregnant at some point in their lives, there's a high likelihood that you, your partner, or a friend may encounter pregnancy discrimination on the job. How's that for a sobering thought?

As you prepare for parenthood, you may find yourself focused on picking a name for your baby or planning your baby shower. But we urge you to save some time, amid all the excitement, to learn how the law protects you as an expecting or new parent and how to fend for yourself where it does not. We've organized the information in this book chronologically to follow the path from pregnancy to parenthood and have tried to highlight key issues and deadlines for you to focus on along the way. We've incorporated stories from real people, whom we met through our legal clinic and advocacy, to bring these issues to life. We have changed all names and some identifying details to protect their privacy and confidentiality. Their experiences also may help prepare you for potential scenarios that may arise and equip you with the tools you need to respond.

As lawyers, we also have to remind you that the information, ideas, and suggestions in this book are not intended to render legal advice. Before following any suggestions contained in this book, you should consult an attorney. Neither we (the authors) nor the publisher shall be liable or responsible for any loss or damage allegedly arising as a consequence of your use or application of any information or suggestions in this book.

We hope the pages that follow will inform and empower you to be an advocate for yourself in the workplace. And in addition to providing this resource, we hope we may inspire you to help improve policies in the United States for working families like yours.

Let's start with a story of two families, one in the United States and one in Sweden:

> **Jenna is from Scranton, Pennsylvania, and she is seven and a half months pregnant. She works as the assistant to the director of human resources at a midsize law firm. Her husband is the manager of a local grocery store. They own a modest home and make ends meet but still feel like they live paycheck to paycheck.**
>
> **Jenna is covered by the Family and Medical Leave Act (FMLA) and can take up to twelve weeks of unpaid family leave in a year. Unfortunately, because her husband's employer has fewer than fifty employees, he is not covered under the act and is not eligible for any family leave. He will have to use his own vacation leave as needed to bond with his new child. Jenna wishes to maximize the time she is able to spend with her baby at home, so she has decided to save as much of her family leave time as she can for after the child's birth. Her frequent prenatal appointments are covered by the FMLA, however, and count toward her total leave time, reducing by nearly two weeks the bonding time she'll have with her baby. And even though Jenna battles fatigue and sickness throughout her pregnancy, she drags herself to work because she doesn't want to use up any more of her time off before the baby arrives.**
>
> **After Jenna has her baby, she begins taking the rest of her twelve weeks of unpaid leave to bond with her**

baby. In the back of her mind, she worries about the fact that she is not earning any income during this time; she worries that she didn't save up enough money in case an emergency should arise. When her newborn is only ten weeks old, Jenna must return to full-time work. She is lucky enough to have a nearby mother-in-law to care for the child while she is at work all day. Otherwise, she would have to find a way to afford day care until her child reaches school age. Even though the child is still a newborn, and the family is comfortably considered middle class, Jenna worries that she will never be able to save up enough money to provide her child with the right opportunities or higher education. She looks for a part-time side job that she can do at home in addition to her full-time job in order to set aside money for the child's future.

•••

Lynn is also seven and a half months pregnant and is from Stockholm, Sweden. She is a waitress at a fine-dining restaurant. Her husband is a real estate agent. They live in a two-bedroom apartment that they rent in the city. They have a secure middle-class lifestyle with relatively little financial insecurity.

Lynn is covered by the Family Benefits laws of Sweden. This means that she and her husband are collectively entitled to take up to 480 days of paid leave per child at 80 percent of their salaries. They can take time off of work for long continuous periods and for single days or parts of days, and they may use their days at any time until the child reaches eight years old or completes his or her first year in school. Because Lynn is less than sixty days away from her due date, she is eligible to use her benefits. She uses her leave time when she is feeling too ill to attend work or when she must attend doctor appointments.

After Lynn has her baby, she and her husband decide to stay home together for the first three months to bond with the baby. After the initial three months, Lynn's husband goes back to work, and Lynn stays at home with the baby for an additional three months. Lynn works out a flexible part-time schedule with her restaurant so that she can go to work while her husband is at home with the baby. She is able to take time off when she needs to while still maintaining a comfortable salary. Further, the Swedish government issues Lynn and her husband a parental allowance to assist in caring for their child. Until the child reaches the age of sixteen, Lynn and her husband get a nontaxable monthly stipend of 1050 Swedish kronor per child, or the equivalent of approximately $155.

Shocked? Jealous? Ready to pack your bags and move to Sweden? The contrast is pretty surprising. As one woman wrote to us:

Unfortunately this country does not realize bringing a new life is also bringing a new citizen, who, if all goes well from the beginning, will be a good student and eventually a productive worker. Why is the beginning of a new life so difficult to cherish?

So how did we get here? Why is US policy so lacking when it comes to supporting pregnancy and parenting?

Picture a scene of a model American family from the 1950s. Dad heads to work every morning with a tip of his hat, leaving Mom at home to care for the children and the household. Dad's employer is probably some big company that offers him a healthy salary generous enough to support a whole family without additional income. Dad's company also probably offers him a wide array of benefits, including health insurance for his wife and kids. Mom does all the hard and mostly invisible domestic work, allowing Dad to stay at the office or factory as long as necessary each day and allowing his employer to rely on him for forty years or so of uninterrupted work. Dad works hard too, but he doesn't have to worry about who will stay home to meet the refrigerator repairman or who will check in on his aging mother or care for his small children. And when he comes home from work, the aroma of a home-cooked meal greets him at the door.

Flash forward to 2014 and you see a very different picture. Today's family may have a mom and dad or one single parent or two parents of the same sex. But no matter what the configuration, parents in today's family are probably all employed and earning wages because few can afford not to. Parents juggle the demands of their jobs with the needs of their families, and the pressure only worsens in a shaky economy, when a job may be here one day but gone the next. With no adult managing the home front full-time, parents must pay (often a lot!) for child care, negotiate who will leave work to pick up a sick child from school, and figure out how on earth they will get a healthy meal on the table each night.

This modern-day juggling act affects families of every size, shape, and income level. Its consequences are far-reaching. The work–family time crunch leads to poor health outcomes for parents and kids, including higher rates of childhood obesity.[3] It drags down wages for working women[4] and those providing care

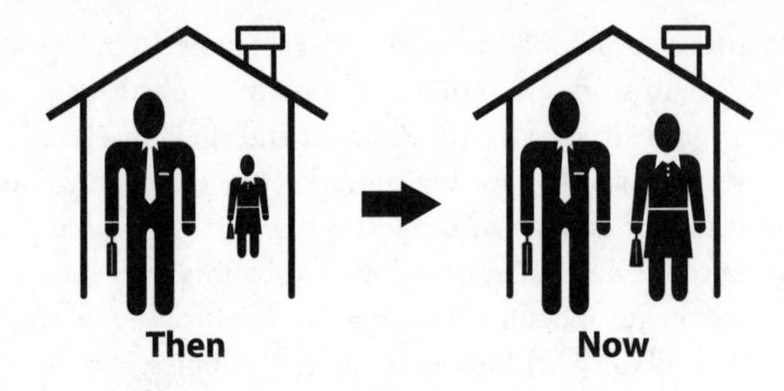

In 1969, women made up only one-third of the workforce in the United States, and more than half of all families had a full-time stay-at-home mom. Today, nearly four in ten moms are the primary breadwinner for their families, and even more are a co-breadwinner.[2]

and perpetuates the gender imbalance and devaluation of domestic work. These consequences hurt us as a society and impact our economy, yet we have few collective solutions to the problem. Here in the United States, we regard this problem as a private issue to be solved on an individual basis, one family and one employee at a time.

Not all countries in the world view family responsibilities this way. Our story of two moms highlights a particularly extreme contrast between Sweden and the United States, but it's not just wealthy Nordic countries that go to bat for their families. Worldwide, 178 countries guarantee some leave with pay to women in connection with childbirth.[5] Seventy-four countries ensure paid paternity leave or the right to paid parental leave for fathers.[6] New mothers in Kazakhstan—a country made famous by Borat—are entitled to more paid maternity leave than mothers in the United States. One hundred twenty-six days of paid leave at 100 percent of their salary, to be exact![7] And our neighbors to the north in

Canada can boast too. Mothers there get seventeen weeks of paid maternity leave, and families may split an additional thirty-five weeks of paid parental leave between the parents as they choose. In Quebec, where fathers get five weeks of nontransferable paternity leave at 70 percent of their earnings, over half of eligible fathers take leave.[8] In contrast, nearly half of new mothers in the United States do not have access to *any* form of paid parental leave.[9]

Maternity leave is only the beginning. When it comes to valuing and supporting the work of caring for families, the United States lags behind the rest of the world in a variety of ways. Our country is one of only a handful that do not guarantee paid sick time for all workers, including time to care for sick family members. In fact, 163 other countries guarantee a minimum number of paid sick days, with many providing a week or more per year for personal health needs.[10] The European Union has sought to eliminate discrimination against part-time workers and improve quality part-time work, but here in the United States part-time workers face discrimination in pay and benefits and are excluded from many labor and employment laws.

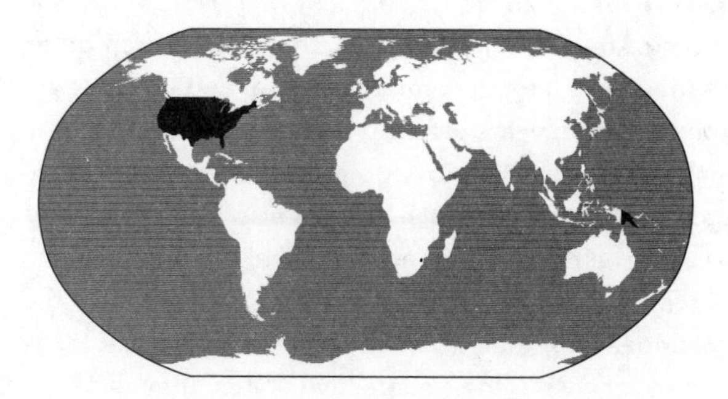

Around the world, 178 countries guarantee paid leave for new mothers. Three countries do not: Swaziland, Papua New Guinea, and the United States.

Dozens of countries provide universal child care at reduced cost to help parents return to work. In 1971, our Congress passed a bill to establish a national day care system in the United States, but President Nixon vetoed the law. More than forty years later, American families are still struggling to find reliable, affordable child care. Wouldn't it be nice to have a high-quality, subsidized child care facility in your neighborhood that is open eleven hours a day? Or if you chose to hire a private nanny instead, to have the government pay her social security, health insurance, and retirement benefits? If this sounds good to you, get ready to brush up on your French and move across the Atlantic!

We tell you all of this not to discourage or depress you (although we admit that sometimes these statistics do bring us down). Rather, we want to show you that it *is* possible for countries to support working families through public policy, and they don't have to be rich or risk their economic prosperity to do it. In fact, here in the United States a few states have started to fill in the gaps left by our meager national policies. Here's an example of just how different the picture can look depending on where you live:

> **Krystal lives in San Francisco, California. Whitney lives in a smaller town in Florida. They don't know each other, but they have a lot in common. Krystal and Whitney are both thirty-two years old, and both work as hostesses in small restaurants. They love going to the beach and relaxing with their friends. Each woman also just had a baby. Because their restaurants are small, neither woman qualifies for the Family and Medical Leave Act (FMLA). The similarities stop there. Considering the rights that these women receive in their respective states, they might as well be living on different planets.**

Whitney stands all day since hostesses aren't allowed to sit on stools at her restaurant. At the end of the day, her feet are so swollen that none of her shoes fit, and she stays in her apartment, exhausted. Whitney finds out that her restaurant doesn't offer maternity leave, and there are no laws to protect her. She gets ten days of paid time off, so she uses all of them after having her baby. Two weeks after giving birth (and after being in labor for twelve hours), she's back at her hostess station. At two weeks old, her baby is too young for day care, and Whitney doesn't have any extended family nearby, so she has to pay $15 per hour to hire a babysitter. She doesn't have time to heal and doesn't even bother trying to breastfeed because she decides it will be too hard to establish in two weeks and too difficult to continue while she's working. She spends $1,700 on formula in the first year, money she doesn't have. Since her hours are unpredictable and her shifts change from week to week, she sometimes can't find a babysitter in time. She asks for a more stable schedule, but her manager won't give her one. She realizes she will have to change professions, so she quits her job. She's incredibly worried about finding a job and having enough money to feed her new baby.

Krystal in California, on the other hand, asks for a stool and is entitled to one by law. One month before giving birth, her doctor puts her on bed rest. Krystal is entitled to disability leave and feels reassured, knowing she can get her job back. She receives state disability insurance payments during this time to pay her bills. She also decides to take six weeks after giving birth under the California Family Rights Act so that she can bond with her new baby. She is paid part of her salary during these

six weeks, so while she is away from work for two and a half months, she is never entirely without income. Krystal breastfeeds successfully and pumps once she gets back to work. Her daughter, at six weeks old, is old enough to go to day care, so Krystal saves money on formula and hiring a babysitter. One day her daughter gets a cold, and Krystal stays home to care for her–in San Francisco, many employees get paid sick days to take care of their sick children. Although Krystal is still working hard to save money and support her family, she doesn't have to worry as much as Whitney does.

We hope that you will keep all of this in mind as we detail the rights you do have under US laws and that you will think about how you might like to see these laws improved, both nationwide and in your home state. If, by the end, you are convinced, we hope you'll join us to bring a better balance to all Americans.

1 CONGRATULATIONS
You're Expecting! Now What?

• POP QUIZ •

(You've probably taken plenty of pregnancy tests already, but we bet some of these answers will surprise you!)

1. **True or false: A woman may be legally fired for carrying a water bottle to stay hydrated when pregnant.**
   True. A court ruled that an employer may not be required by federal law to accommodate the needs of a healthy pregnant woman (i.e., one without any disabling or complicating condition). This is a true story!

2. **You announce your pregnancy to your boss, who says, "As soon as you start showing, you'll have to go on disability because we can't have you looking like that in front of our customers." Is this illegal?**
   Yes. You cannot be forced out on leave if you are able to do your job. Opinions of customers are not a valid excuse for discrimination.

3. **You are offered a job, but before accepting, you ask about the company's maternity leave policy because you are planning a pregnancy. The company abruptly withdraws the job offer. Is this illegal?**
   Probably. Proving this form of discrimination requires evidence of intent and is never a sure thing, but this is pretty suggestive of unlawful bias based on pregnancy.

It's official. You peed on a stick and saw the sign. You are about to enter the next phase of your life. But now what?

Finding out you are pregnant should be an occasion for celebration, but it can also lead to anxiety or, even worse, unfair treatment on the job. You may start asking yourself questions: How and when should I tell my boss about my pregnancy? What if I need to take time off for prenatal appointments or morning sickness? What should I do if I think I'm not being treated fairly at work because of my pregnancy or impending parenthood? What are my legal rights as a pregnant woman, and which laws cover me?

This chapter aims to answer these questions and others you may encounter during your pregnancy. We start with a discussion of how to break the news of your pregnancy at work, including how to handle interview questions about pregnancy. Then we review the Pregnancy Discrimination Act and how it does (and sometimes doesn't) protect you at work. In addition to describing the law, we offer tips on how to handle situations not technically covered by the law. We move on to discuss how the law may help you get a job modification to accommodate your pregnancy. Finally we tackle the topics of illness and prenatal care and whether you are entitled to any time off for your health needs while pregnant. Ready? Let's get started.

INTERVIEWING WHILE PREGNANT

What if you are trying to nail down a new job while pregnant? How do you handle that? First of all, you are not required to disclose your pregnancy to a potential employer, even if your bulging belly gives it away. You may decide to address the issue head-on and confront any assumptions your interviewer may have about your ability or intentions. But that's up to you. Generally speaking, potential employers should not ask you about your pregnancy or family plans during the interview process. Such questions could indicate discrimination. Although not all questions are illegal, they may be if directed at only some people (i.e., women) and not others. For example, an interviewer can't ask only women if they have children, and not ask the same question of men. Also, if you live in a state with more protective laws, certain questions may be expressly prohibited. (Check the state-by-state guide on page 201 for more information.)

If you are suspicious of an interview question, first make a mental note, so that you can jot it down after the interview for your records. (Some helpful advice: it's always a good idea to take notes with dates of anything that smells fishy.) Then, instead of calling out your interviewer, try to address his or her underlying concerns while indicating that you don't think the question is appropriate.

Here's a hypothetical example:

Christina is interviewing for a job as the buyer for women's apparel at a large nationwide clothing store. She has excellent credentials and nearly seven years of experience in the business. Her current position, as an assistant to a fashion designer, has required her to work late nights and travel extensively. She recently got married and is looking for a position that will allow her more control over her schedule in anticipation of starting a family.

INTERVIEWER: So, I see that you're working for Bob Duran. That's a plum job! Why would you want to leave?

CHRISTINA: Working with Bob has been a tremendous opportunity for me, but I'm looking for a different kind of experience at this point.

INTERVIEWER: And why is this job the answer?

CHRISTINA: I am eager to take on new responsibilities and apply my proven skill set to this position as a buyer, where I can have more creative control than as an assistant. I learned a ton from Bob, but it's time to break out on my own.

INTERVIEWER: He does cast a large shadow . . . So are you willing to put in Bob Duran–type hours in this job? We really need someone who will put in 110 percent. Our last buyer was great, but she had a baby and wanted to work part-time, and that just wasn't going to work.

CHRISTINA: Well, I am certainly willing to work hard and get the job done.

INTERVIEWER: But you also recently got married, right? Do you plan on having a baby soon?

CHRISTINA: I am really just enjoying being a newlywed at this point. My career is a major priority for me, and I am fully prepared to do an excellent job in this position no matter what my home life looks like. I have a solid work ethic and am excited to contribute to the team.

You've done your best interview jujitsu to deflect interview questions about your pregnancy or family plans, but you still don't get the job. What now?

First, you should know what the law prohibits. An employer cannot refuse to hire you because you are pregnant and may not consider your pregnancy or possible pregnancy when deciding whether to hire you. The law entitles you to be judged on your capacity to do the job. For example, an employer can't base his or her decision not to hire you on the assumption that, as a pregnant woman, you might have difficulty doing your job at some point or because he or she thinks customers would not want to deal with a pregnant woman. Similarly, an employer may not refuse to hire you based on the assumption that because you have (or will soon have) small children, you'll be a distracted and unreliable employee. However, the law allows an employer to refuse to hire you if you cannot perform the major functions necessary to the job. If you disclose your pregnancy and indicate that you will need an extended leave during a time when the employer needs all hands on deck or indicate that you will not be able to work the required hours for the job, an employer might legally consider that information in refusing to hire you.

Think back to your interview and any other comments or interactions you encountered during your application process. If you have a strong sense that an employer improperly considered your pregnancy in the decision not to hire you, you may want to reach out to a lawyer for specific advice regarding your situation. It can be hard to prove that discrimination was at the heart of a decision not to hire you, but a lawyer can help you determine your best options.

What if you are offered a job, and the employer doesn't know about your pregnancy? Again, you are under no obligation to disclose your pregnancy. In fact, if you do tell your new employer and the employer withdraws the offer, that alone could be illegal, and you can seek help from a lawyer. However, you may want to discuss your situation openly before accepting the job if you are concerned about how your pregnancy might interact with the job responsibilities. Also, keep in mind that you could risk the goodwill of your new boss if you keep this information to yourself and then announce, shortly after starting the job, that you are pregnant and will need time off. Assuming you don't want to start your new job off on the wrong foot, honesty might be the best policy.

CAN WE TALK? BREAKING THE NEWS OF YOUR PREGNANCY AT WORK

Many women we talk to say how afraid they are of telling their boss about their pregnancy. This fear is real and often based on true stories of women who lost their jobs after announcing their pregnancy. Here are two of them:

> **I received a FedEx envelope at my door one morning; the owner of the gallery had been informed (from a colleague) that I had recently learned I was pregnant with my second child, [and] he felt that was an opportune time to "dismiss" me from my position as I would not be, as the letter of dismissal stated, "able to fulfill [my] obligations as Gallery Director."**

> **I got fired from my job at a private ambulance exactly one week after telling my boss I was pregnant. I was almost five months along. He immediately started looking for a reason to fire me. And he finally created one. You know what he did? He took the power stretcher off my truck and replaced it with a manual one (the kind you have to heave up to get it up/down/in/out the ambulance). I saw the power stretcher in the garage, unused and working perfectly, so I put it back on my truck, and used it to transport three patients. He then fired me for switching equipment without his permission . . . The**

icing on the cake? He fired me one week before I was eligible for unemployment.

These stories are horrible and, unfortunately, not uncommon. Although there is no guarantee that your employer will welcome your pregnancy news, we want to offer some general thoughts and tips as you approach this important conversation.

When to Tell

After you've shared your happy news with your family and close friends, you may wonder when you should tell your colleagues and your boss that you are expecting. Unless you need to request time off for pregnancy-related illness, there are no real legal deadlines for notifying your employer until late in your pregnancy, when you might need to request leave thirty days in advance of taking off for childbirth (see chapter 2 for more information). Still, at some point before that it will be apparent to those around you that your body is changing. Ultimately, the decision of when to tell others about your pregnancy is yours. That being said, there are a few things you should consider when making your decision.

As you have probably heard, the most uncertain period of your pregnancy is the first trimester, when miscarriages are more common. You may not want to give notice of your pregnancy at work too early, only to confront the pain of sharing the news of a miscarriage with your employer too. Keeping the secret to yourself for a while can also give you time to do some initial digging about your employer's leave policies and some research about state and federal laws that might apply to you.

On the other hand, you may find it hard to stay quiet when you are exhausted, are feeling nauseated, and could really benefit from the support of your colleagues. Telling select colleagues early may allow you to talk openly with those you trust and find out how your employer has handled others' pregnancies and leaves of absence before yours. Telling your boss can help you avoid health risks for you and your baby if you work in a job with safety hazards and will give your boss more time to digest the news, adjust to any restrictions that your pregnancy poses, and prepare for your leave. Sharing your news early also may generate goodwill from your boss (a valuable commodity!), who will certainly appreciate the extra time to plan around your maternity leave.

If your employer has a human resources department, you might consider telling them about your pregnancy first, before telling your supervisor. They may know more about the company's policies than your boss does. However, be aware that the HR department's first priority is your employer, not you. The department is not there to protect your interests.

It all boils down to how you feel about your work environment. If you feel comfortable and confident that your employer will take your news well, then by all means feel free to share as soon as you want. Beware, however, that a previously supportive supervisor can turn nasty once you've announced your pregnancy. We hear stories like this all the time through our hotline. If you already suspect that your news may not be well received, don't feel pressure to disclose your pregnancy before you are ready. Take your time!

What to Say

When you do decide to tell your boss about your pregnancy, keep in mind that your happy news may be a source of stress for him or her. Despite the fact that the majority of working women return to work after giving birth, and most very successfully, some employers still fear that pregnancy and motherhood will mean losing a dedicated employee. To ease any worry your boss may have, reassure him or her that you are committed to your job and that you plan to return to work after the baby arrives. Offer your help in planning for your absence—for example, in planning who will cover your work while you are gone and how/if you will stay in touch while you are on leave. Be prepared for a conversation about maternity leave, and do your homework so that you know what the law guarantees and what you want to request from your employer (see chapter 2 for more information on the law, and take a look at the chapter 2 resources page for templates and tips to guide you in your negotiation). This will help you to negotiate the best possible outcome for you and your family.

So far, we've been assuming that you want to return to work after your baby arrives. But what if you don't want to? It can be hard to anticipate how you will feel post-baby. The idea of caring for a dependent little person while also going to work every day may seem daunting in those early weeks. But you might also crave some independence and the benefits that work provides (not the least of which is money!). Give yourself time to make this decision so that you don't close any doors on yourself unnecessarily.

DID HE REALLY JUST SAY THAT?
CONFRONTING DISCRIMINATION AT WORK

Susan worked diligently for a small magazine for over a year, traveling and spending extensive time away from her fiancé. As her wedding date neared, her boss started asking whether her fiancé earned a good living

and about her plans for starting a family. He even threatened, "You better not get pregnant on your honeymoon because we need you here." Her coworkers also repeatedly told her she should not get pregnant on her honeymoon. Despite her excellent performance reviews, Susan was fired just a few weeks before she left on her honeymoon.

Even though discrimination based on pregnancy has been illegal for thirty-five years, bias against pregnant women is still common today. Some of this bias is tied to assumptions about child-care responsibilities and a pregnant woman's future dedication to work (see chapter 4 for more). But some is just bias based on pregnancy itself. This kind of discrimination can have serious consequences, forcing a woman out of her job or into a lower-paying position with fewer benefits and opportunities. We want to help you know how to identify illegal discrimination and learn what you can do to protect yourself should it happen to you.

Keep in mind that even if your employer does something illegal under the law, litigation may not be the most effective strategy for you. For example, it may be too hard to prove that your suspicions are right if you don't have enough evidence to show discrimination. Or you may not want to jeopardize your career in a particular field by filing a claim against your current employer. Or maybe you just don't want to deal with the time and expense of litigation. Knowing your rights up front may help you to avoid the worst-case scenario of litigation and keep you healthy and earning a paycheck. We hope the information we offer here can help empower you to stand up for yourself or seek help as soon as you sense a problem. Prevention is often the best medicine.

The Pregnancy Discrimination Act in a Nutshell

WHAT?

The Pregnancy Discrimination Act (PDA) is a federal law that prohibits unfair treatment of women because of their pregnancy. It requires employers to treat women affected by pregnancy, childbirth, or related medical conditions the same as other job applicants or employees who are similarly limited in their ability to work (such as someone who has an injured back, for example).

WHO?

If you work for a private employer with fifteen or more employees, you are protected by the PDA. You are also covered if you work for state or local government. The law protects you as a job applicant from unlawful discrimination in hiring decisions as well. If you work for a private employer with fewer than fifteen employees, check our guide at the end of this book to see whether your state has a sex discrimination law that applies to smaller workplaces.

WHEN?

The PDA kicks in when you become pregnant, but it may also protect you when you are not yet pregnant or have already given birth. For example, if your boss is hostile or unaccommodating because she or he thinks you are pregnant or thinks you may become pregnant, that could be illegal. The PDA might also protect you after you come back from maternity leave, depending on the circumstances.

HOW?

The law prohibits your employer from discriminating against you in any aspect of employment, which includes hiring, firing, pay, job assignments, promotions, layoffs, training, fringe benefits such as leave and health insurance, and any other term or condition of employment. Harassment based on pregnancy is also unlawful. Your employer also cannot force you to take a leave from work if you are still willing and able to do your job. Your employer must treat you the same as other employees who temporarily can't do their jobs—for example, if someone with a broken hand is given modified work or someone recovering from heart surgery is given unpaid leave, you as a pregnant woman or brand-new mom are entitled to the same treatment.

WHY?

Discrimination based on sex was outlawed across the United States in 1964, but women were still routinely fired or expected to quit when they became pregnant. In 1978, Congress amended the Civil Rights Act of 1964 to clarify the law and guarantee equal opportunity for pregnant women and new mothers. The PDA is a minimum requirement, however, which means employers *can* offer more generous leave options to pregnant women than they offer other employees. State laws may also offer more protections than the PDA, so be sure to check out the state-by-state guide for more information.

What's Right and What's Wrong?

What is pregnancy discrimination?

1. An employer may not discriminate against you in hiring, firing, or any other terms, conditions, or privileges of your employment because of pregnancy, childbirth, or related medical conditions. What does that mean? Basically, an employer can't take negative action against you at work, or in the decision to hire you, because of your pregnancy,

because of your upcoming or recent childbirth, or because of any pregnancy- or childbirth-related medical conditions. Here's a hypothetical example of illegal discrimination:

Jackie worked as a hostess at a popular and pricey cocktail lounge. When she told her boss that she was expecting a baby, he thanked her for her service and told her she was longer needed. In his words, "We can't have you lumbering about with a tray full of cocktails. Our customers expect a more refined experience."

2. Also, as we discussed earlier in this chapter, pregnant women and those affected by childbirth or related medical conditions must be treated the same as other workers who are similarly unable to work. Here's another hypothetical example:

   Alisha worked as a dental hygienist. When she got pregnant, her boss told her the office didn't have a maternity leave policy, and she would have to return to work as soon as she used up all her sick and vacation time. Alisha found out that a former employee had been allowed to take unpaid leave for a month after surgery for breast cancer. Alisha should be allowed to take a similar unpaid leave after giving birth.

Does that mean my employer can't fire me while I'm pregnant?

No. The law does not automatically protect you while you are pregnant. Your employer can still fire you or treat you badly for other reasons, just not because of your pregnancy. So if your work performance or attendance suffers during pregnancy, you are not protected from any discipline at work just because you are pregnant. Your boss can discipline you for those things, as long as she or he applies the same standards to you as to nonpregnant employees. In the United States, we generally have an "at will" employment system, meaning your employer can fire you at any time for any reason (because he or she doesn't like your haircut, because you were late once, because your boss has decided he or she just doesn't like you, etc.). There are a few exceptions—namely, your employer can't fire you for discriminatory reasons, like if he or she found out that you were a Muslim or that you were pregnant.

Ever since I announced my pregnancy, my employer has been making my life miserable. My boss docks me a day's pay for every time I come in late because of morning sickness and for each time I have a prenatal appointment with my doctor. He has repeatedly made nasty remarks about my pregnancy. Is this illegal? I'm seriously thinking of quitting because I just can't take it anymore.
Harassment based on sex that is severe enough to create a hostile work environment is illegal. If your employer is harassing you because of your pregnancy, that is harassment based on sex and, if serious enough, may be unlawful. If the situation is so bad as to be unbearable, you may be experiencing something called "constructive discharge." That means if you quit, you may have a claim against your employer because you were forced to do so, even if your boss never formally fired you.

I recently suffered my fourth miscarriage in a year, and my employer advised me to stop trying to get pregnant for a while, since it was obviously not working out. She told me I was missing

ADVERSE ACTIONS

In order to have a legal claim, you need to experience an "adverse action" or negative consequence as a result of discrimination. What does that mean? Let's say that your boss says some inappropriate things about your pregnancy, but her or his comments have no real impact on your job. They're not severe enough to amount to harassment, and you are able to continue working, take your maternity leave, and return to your job without incident. In this case, even though you feel offended and may have experienced some discrimination, there's been no adverse action, so you are unlikely to have a claim for relief. What is an adverse action? Here are some examples.

After announcing your pregnancy at work, the following happens:

- Your boss cuts your hours, even though you never asked for reduced hours.
- You suddenly start receiving poor performance reviews.
- Your boss targets you for unsuitable or dangerous work.
- Your boss tells you to train others to do your job and transfers you into a lower-paying position.

too much time from work to recover and did not consider me for a promotion because of all of my absences. Is this illegal?

Possibly. The PDA protects you from discrimination based on pregnancy and related medical conditions, which includes miscarriage and abortion. Your employer's first statement alone may not be enough to prove discrimination, but when viewed together with her decision to deny you a promotion, it is probably enough to suggest unlawful behavior. If you have a pregnancy-related disability, including a high-risk pregnancy, you also may be protected by the Americans with Disabilities Act or a similar local law (see the section below—Workplace Accommodations for Complicated or Difficult Pregnancies—for more information).

I recently found out that I was carrying a fetus with severe genetic mutations. My partner and I decided to terminate the pregnancy, but my health care plan is refusing to reimburse me for the medical costs. Is this illegal?

No. Although it is true that any employer-provided health insurance must cover expenses for pregnancy-related conditions on the same basis as costs for other medical conditions, the PDA does not require expenses arising from abortion to be covered, except where the life of the mother is in danger.

I told my immediate supervisor I was pregnant, but I haven't discussed it with our boss yet. When I told my supervisor, she said I better be sure not to make her life hard by taking time off for sickness or doctor's appointments. Is this pregnancy discrimination?

It could be pregnancy discrimination even though it was only your supervisor who threatened you. A lawyer could help you figure out the answer in a specific case. But it's important to cover all your bases by telling a higher-up boss or your human resources

UNEMPLOYMENT INSURANCE

If you do decide to quit your job, keep in mind that whether or not you can receive unemployment benefits will depend on how you leave. This is important because unemployment benefits can provide critical income to your family while you are out of work. To be eligible for unemployment benefits, you must have lost your job through no fault of your own, and be ready, willing, and able to work. The standards vary from state to state, but generally, you will not be eligible for benefits if you lose your job because of a personal choice. Quitting is generally seen as your choice and therefore your "fault." Constructive discharge, or being effectively forced out of your job, is generally not considered your fault and should not disqualify you from unemployment insurance benefits. The law also may allow for certain exceptions where you can quit with what's called "good cause." For example, if you quit because of a medical reason related to your pregnancy, you may be able to collect benefits, even though you quit. If your job is high-stress and you have a high-risk pregnancy that is made riskier by the stress of your job, and your doctor advises you to stop working, you may be eligible for unemployment benefits, even if you are the one to call it quits. Similarly, if your employer refuses to allow you time off to attend prenatal medical appointments, you might have good cause to quit. Since the rules for unemployment insurance differ depending on the state where you live, check with a local expert before you take the plunge.

department about your pregnancy—and by telling them about any discrimination you feel you are experiencing. It's also worth noting that women can be biased just as much as men; when it comes to discrimination, it is irrelevant whether a boss, supervisor, or human resource manager is male or female.

It's common knowledge at the hotel where I work that pregnant employees will be asked to go home to "rest" when they start showing and will probably not be hired back after they give birth. Do I really have any rights if this is my employer's policy?

Yes. The fact that your employer routinely forces pregnant women out of their jobs does not make it any more legal. You may want to enlist the support of an attorney or call a legal hotline or community group to get some advice before you try to discuss the issue with your employer.

Does the PDA guarantee maternity leave?

No. The PDA does not guarantee you any time off related to childbirth and does not protect your job while you are giving birth or recovering from delivery. (Read chapter 2 to see whether you might be entitled to job-protected time off under the Family and Medical Leave Act, and keep an eye out for interpretations of the Americans with Disabilities Act that might include recovery from childbirth as a disabling condition entitled to accommodation.) The PDA requires only that pregnant women be treated the same as other employees. This means that if your employer grants leave for employees with temporary disabilities, it must grant you some leave too for recovery from childbirth. But if your employer does not grant any temporary leave or sick leave of any kind for anyone, it does not have to provide leave for you related to your pregnancy. (If you work for an employer without any leave policy, you may still be entitled to some maternity or pregnancy disability leave under state law. Check out our state-by-state guide for more specifics about your state's laws.)

On the other hand, the law does allow employers to do more for pregnant women if they want. The requirement of equal treatment prevents employers from treating pregnant women *worse* than other employees, but it doesn't prohibit them from treating them better. For example, an employer can offer pregnancy disability leave to women, calling it maternity leave, and not offer the same to men. However, if an employer offers leave for purposes of bonding with a new child (not for recovery from the physical demands of childbirth), it must offer that to all parents, not just birth mothers.

How can I tell what type of leave my employer provides?

Look at your employee handbook. Check to see how birth mothers, temporarily disabled individuals, new parents, and those dealing with a family emergency are treated. If there is no employee handbook, or you are confused, you can ask around and find out who has previously been given leave and why.

Can my employer force me onto disability leave?

As long as you can do your job, you cannot be forced out. You must be allowed to work as long as you are able to do the work. The flip side of this is that if you cannot do the work required of your job, and your employer does not help out anyone else with similar limitations, you may be let go or forced onto unpaid leave. If you are forced out or are absent as the result of a pregnancy-related condition, but you then recover and are able to work again, your employer cannot require you to remain on leave until your baby is born. You must be allowed back to work.

What if I am forced onto disability and because of that don't have enough hours to be eligible for the FMLA?

Aside from a potential PDA violation (as discussed previously), you may be dealing with a violation of the Family and Medical Leave Act. We talk more about the FMLA in chapter 2, including how many hours you must work to be eligible for time off. For now, you should know that if your employer is covered by the FMLA, your boss must not interfere with your rights under the law. Forcing you out on disability in order to prevent you from working the hours you need to qualify for FMLA leave could

TIME-OUT FOR OUTRAGE!

Fact: a woman will not be able to work for a bit of time while she is in labor and recovering from childbirth. Fact: many women in the United States cannot take even minimal time off to welcome a baby without the risk of losing their jobs. Depending on which state they call home, women who work for smaller companies (those with under fifty employees) often have no right to time off to give birth. This is particularly true for women in low-wage jobs that lack basic benefits such as paid sick time, which could be used for childbirth. Contrast this with the United Kingdom, where all female employees are guaranteed up to fifty-two weeks of maternity leave by law and new mothers have to take at least two weeks of time off after giving birth! It's enough to raise your blood pressure, right?

potentially amount to illegal interference with your rights. If this has happened to you, consult with a lawyer or workers' rights advocate about your options.

Does the Law Cover Me?

Does the law protect me if I'm not pregnant yet or anymore?

It should. Some "savvy" employers think that they can just delay firing a pregnant woman until after she returns from maternity leave, and they will be cleared of all wrongdoing. Not so fast, sneaky sexists! If you can show that you were treated unfairly *because of* your pregnancy, childbirth, or some related medical condition, the law should protect you *even if* you were not actually pregnant at the time of the mistreatment. This is an area of the law where courts are still ironing out the details. For example, some courts have found that the PDA protects from discrimination women who are on maternity leave and those who have just returned to work from maternity leave. (The FMLA, which we discuss in chapter 2, may also apply in this situation.) Here's an example:

> **A woman who worked as a paralegal at a law firm for over fifteen years, who received glowing reviews all along, was terminated eleven days after she returned from maternity leave. One of the firm partners noted that she "had been out quite a bit the last nine months." Another paralegal at the firm was also fired shortly after returning from maternity leave, after another of the firm's partners suggested that her pregnancy created "the perfect opportunity to get rid of her."**

Other courts have held that the PDA prohibits discrimination against women on the basis of their ability to become pregnant and that the law prohibits an employer from firing a woman for undergoing IVF treatments. Here's a real story from a recent case:

> **Elira worked as a server at a restaurant in a touristy area of New York City. The female servers and bartenders were encouraged to flirt with patrons. Elira had a friendly relationship with her supervisors and shared with them her hopes of becoming a mother. However, the day after she announced that she was moving from the evaluation and diagnostic phase of IVF to the treatment stage, she was fired.**[11]

Not only are prepregnancy conditions covered, but discrimination against a woman because of her postpartum depression is also prohibited by the PDA (and the ADA, as discussed previously; see the section below—Workplace Accommodations for Complicated or Difficult Pregnancies—for more information). Definitely don't rule out the possibility that the law may cover you just because you are not pregnant at the time you perceive discrimination. If you find yourself in this situation, you should seek legal advice. Also, be sure to write down the details of what your employer says to you, or what you overhear, while it's still fresh in your mind. And if a colleague tells you about comments he or she overheard, write that down too. The key will be tying what your employer did to your pregnancy or childbirth.

Does the law protect me if I am an independent contractor/ freelancer/self-employed?

No. Unfortunately, the definition of "employee" under the PDA does not include independent contractors (whom the law treats the same as freelancers and those who are self-employed). That being said, plenty of employers improperly call their employees independent contractors to avoid complying with the laws that protect employees. So don't assume you are not protected by the PDA just because the place where you work denies you an employee benefit plan, pays you by the hour, or treats you like an independent contractor for tax purposes. You could still be an employee, especially if you do not have a great deal of control over how and when you do your work. If you have any doubt about your status and the legal protections you may be missing out on, it's a good idea to consult an attorney. And even if you are an independent contractor, you still may be able to seek justice under the common law (e.g., by claiming breach of contract) or your local law.

Does the law protect me if I am an undocumented immigrant?
Yes. The PDA does not let your employer off the hook just because you are an undocumented immigrant. However, being undocumented may affect what a court can require your employer to do if you are seeking to get your job back or to be paid for the time after which you were fired. You should seek the support of a lawyer and/or a workers' rights community organization if you are worried about the consequences of your immigration status.

After being passed over for a few key assignments, I told my supervisor that I felt like she was treating me unfairly because I am pregnant, and then, two days later, she took away my flexible work schedule. Is this illegal?
It could well be. The Pregnancy Discrimination Act prohibits retaliation for exercising your rights, or complaining about potential violations of those rights, under the law. Retaliation usually hap-

pens close in time to the protected activity, and includes adverse actions (punishments) by an employer that could have dissuaded a reasonable worker from making or supporting a charge of discrimination. According to the Supreme Court, this could include taking away a flexible work schedule from a mother with young children.

What Can I Do?

I'm six months pregnant, and no one will hire me. I think it's because my pregnancy is showing, but what can I do about it?

As we said earlier, it is illegal to not hire someone because she is pregnant. However, proving this might be difficult. If your interviewer did not acknowledge your pregnancy, then he or she can simply say that the company didn't hire you because there was a more qualified applicant or that he or she got along with the other applicant better in the interview. In a tough economy, there will probably be no shortage of applicants, so proving a discriminatory intent can be difficult. However, talk to a lawyer; there might be something that can be done.

News of my pregnancy did not go over well with my employer, and I'm nervous that they might try to force me out of my job. What should I do?

The first thing to do if you suspect some kind of pregnancy bias is keep careful records of your conversations with your boss or other supervisors at work. Hopefully, the situation never comes to this, but if you do find yourself trying to prove discrimination down the road, this evidence will be helpful to support your case. When possible, correspond by email, and confirm conversations that way, so that you can be sure to have as much in writing as you can. Be sure to keep your files private, and do not store them on your work computer. Try talking to your boss and letting her or him know that despite your pregnancy, you want to stay on the job and will be able to work just as you did before. If your boss starts threatening you with termination, you could even let her or him know that it is illegal to fire someone because of pregnancy, but tread carefully. If you are ultimately fired or demoted, or you experience some other negative decision by your employer, you will want to seek some legal advice to assess the strength of your claims and your options for taking action.

My employer fired me a week after I announced my pregnancy but said it was because of tardiness. I have been late a few times in the last year, but my boss never mentioned it being a problem before! I think she just doesn't want a pregnant woman in the store, but I don't know if I can prove what's in her head. Is there anything I can do?

Yes, you should talk to a lawyer about your specific situation, but you might have a pregnancy discrimination claim. As in much of life, the timing here is key. If you were fired shortly after announcing your pregnancy, that could be evidence of a discriminatory motive. What should you do? If filing a lawsuit seems like too much for you to handle, don't throw in the towel! Sometimes a lawyer or other advocate can send a simple letter telling your employer that its actions were illegal, which could convince your boss to change her mind and rehire you.

I think my employer may have illegally fired me a few years ago, but I wasn't ready at the time to fight them because I was dealing with the stress of a high-risk pregnancy and then a new baby. Is it too late to file a claim?

The PDA requires that before you file a claim in court, you first try to resolve your dispute before the Equal Employment Opportunity Commission (EEOC) or a state agency that enforces the law. The EEOC is a federal government agency that enforces discrimination laws. The time limit for filing a charge with the EEOC is 180 days (around six months), although it may be longer if you live in a state that also enforces an antidiscrimination law similar to the PDA.

If the discrimination you suspect didn't result in the loss of your job but did impact your pay, you may be able to take advantage of a longer deadline for filing your claim. In 2009, Congress passed a law to address the case of Lilly Ledbetter, who worked for Goodyear Tire for almost twenty years before discovering that she had been paid less than her male counterparts that whole time. She sued Goodyear, but the Supreme Court ruled against her, saying that she had missed the 180-day deadline for filing her claim. The court said that the first time she was paid less because of gender discrimination marked the start of her time clock, and since that was years before she filed her claim, she was out of luck. Congress passed the Lilly Ledbetter Fair Pay Act to fix this problem; now, with every new paycheck you get that is tainted by discrimination, your clock for filing a claim resets.

Even if you are too late to file a claim, you can still make your voice heard. You can contact a women's rights organization or community group that cares about pregnancy discrimination and share your story so that they may use it in their fight for better laws (you can always contact our organization at babygate@abetterbalance.org). You also may want to contact your state attorney general's office and report any discrimination you suspect. Sometimes, employers can be repeat offenders, and the attorney general's office may want to investigate a problem employer, even after the time limit for filing a claim has passed. Pursuing justice outside of the legal system might not help you get your job or pay back, but it can have a big impact on laws and policies that will protect you and other women in the future.

STAYING HEALTHY AND EMPLOYED: WORKPLACE ACCOMMODATIONS FOR PREGNANCY

Alexandra worked for two years as the office manager in a small doctor's office. Her relationship with the doctor was generally strained, but in the months after she announced her pregnancy, it got progressively worse. The doctor did not allow Alexandra to take a lunch break or use any paid time off for her prenatal appointments, so when she had to visit the doctor, she had to take a full day off work without pay. Halfway into her pregnancy, the doctor told Alexandra that he was demoting her and cutting her pay and instructed her to train another employee to take over her responsibilities. Shortly thereafter, he fired her. Alexandra's boss told her that he should have fired her on the spot once she informed him she was pregnant and that any reference he might give her would depend on how she handled her termination.

I was pregnant and had horrible morning sickness (my doctor was going to hospitalize me–it was that bad) and was running to throw up every twenty minutes. [My bosses] seemed like they would be accommodating, having a separate place for women to pump, but they told me [that] they would only give me one extra fifteen-minute break (that I couldn't split [it] up into fif-

teen one-minute breaks to get sick; I could only take one a day) AND I had to email someone and get permission before I could use it . . . I was fired when one day I was driving to work and threw up in the car and was late to work because I had to change and clean up . . . I called to let them know, and they told me to come in covered in puke if I had to, but if I was late, [not to] bother coming in.

Unfortunately, we hear lots of stories like these—pregnant women who experience unfair treatment at work after announcing their pregnancies. Although we hope you are fortunate enough to have a boss who is understanding and eager to help, we realize this may not be the case. Even those who have good relationships with their employers sometimes see those relationships sour once the news is out.

Workplace Accommodations for Complicated or Difficult Pregnancies

We hope that you are blessed with an easy pregnancy and that you glow right through your due date! But you may find yourself, like many women, facing unexpected complications related to your pregnancy. These could range from severe morning sickness to a diagnosis of preeclampsia or some other condition. If this does happen, keep in mind that you may have additional rights under federal, state, and local disability laws designed to help people with limitations stay on the job. If you have a disability under the law, you can seek what is called a "reasonable accommodation" from your employer—that is, some change to your workplace or work schedule that allows you to continue working despite your condition, such as the option to work from home. Such accommodations are required unless they impose an "undue hardship" on your employer's business. For example, a particular business may not be able to function with someone working part-time or may not be able to afford special equipment that someone with a disability might need. If that is the case, then the business is not required to make these accommodations.

Recent amendments to the Americans with Disabilities Act have made it easier for a wider range of people and disabilities to qualify for protection, including women with pregnancy-related disorders. For example, a woman diagnosed with gestational diabetes may be covered by the law and entitled to reasonable accommodations from her employer. Let's say this woman works as a cashier at a big-box store and usually is allowed only one meal break at lunchtime. With her diagnosis, she may qualify as having a disability (even if only temporarily) under the law and be entitled to more frequent meal breaks. These minor changes to her schedule may allow her to keep working in spite of her condition, whereas without them she might be forced onto unpaid leave or be forced to quit her job. It's important to remember, though, that the law doesn't guarantee you the exact reasonable accommodation that you request, just any accommodation that will let you do your job. It's up to the employer to decide which accommodation might be best.

We hear from lots of women who have high-risk pregnancies these days, and many of them also may be protected under the recent amendments to the Americans with Disabilities Act. This is an area of law that is still being ironed out, but the Equal Employment Opportunity Commission has been encouraged to issue some clarifying guidance on this topic.[12] Even if you don't think of yourself as disabled or high-risk, the Americans with Disabilities

Act or a local disability law could still cover you. If you have back pain, spotting, nausea, fatigue, hypertension, migraines, or other conditions that are exacerbated by your pregnancy, for example, then you might be protected, depending on other factors (check with a lawyer and take a look at our full list on page 184).

Not only do you have to have one of these issues to be protected by the law, but your condition also has to affect your daily life in some way (the legal term is that it must "substantially limit a major lift activity"). For example, the EEOC has clarified that "someone with an impairment resulting in a twenty-pound lifting restriction that lasts or is expected to last for several months is substantially limited in the major life activity of lifting." Also, to be protected by the law, you have to tell your employer about the specific problem you are facing, not just the fact that you are pregnant. Mention the condition in writing just to be sure, but read our caveats about doctor's notes in the next section. We don't want to get your hopes up, because as we said, this is a very uncertain area of the law, but we think there is an opportunity to expand rights to more workers who need them right now. If you find yourself in need of a minor adjustment at work because of your pregnancy, we really encourage you to seek legal advice.

The Americans with Disabilities Act in a Nutshell

WHAT?

The Americans with Disabilities Act (ADA) is a federal law that bans discrimination against people with disabilities in employment and other areas. The law defines a disability as a physical or mental impairment that substantially limits a major life activity. This means that those with pregnancy-related disabilities, such as gestational diabetes, are probably covered by the ADA. However, normal pregnancy is not covered.

WHO?

You are protected by the ADA if you work for a private employer with fifteen or more employees. You are also covered if you work for the state or local government. If you work for a private employer with fewer than fifteen employees, check our state-by-state guide to see if your state has a disability discrimination law that applies to smaller workplaces.

WHEN?

This law kicks in whenever your employer knows about any qualifying limitation that you have. The law also applies if your employer thinks that you have a disability, even if you don't, or if you are associated with someone with a disability, such as a child with special needs.

HOW?

The law does not just protect against discrimination in hiring, training, pay, and other employment privileges. It also requires employers to accommodate employees with disabilities so that they can do their jobs. Reasonable accommodations might include modifying equipment or reassigning someone to an open job position that might suit her or his needs better. You could try to get a part-time schedule, for example, although your employer does not have to do anything that would come at great cost to the business. Reasonable accommodations are not required, however, for workers who have an association with a person with a disability. This means that the parent of a child with severe asthma, for example, would not be entitled to an alternate work schedule to accommodate caregiving responsibilities to his or her child.

WHY?

Congress passed this law in 1990 to eliminate discrimination against people with disabilities. Congress passed amendments to the law in 2008 because Congress did not like how the Supreme Court had limited the law. The new amendments ensure that the law will cover many more people.

The Americans with Disabilities Act (ADA) also requires an interactive process, where your employer has to consider your individual situation and try, in good faith, to find a solution to help you stay on the job. Many states and cities have laws that mirror the ADA but that are even more inclusive than the federal law. In New York State and New York City, for example, failing to engage an employee in an interactive process could be a violation of the law in and of itself. Local laws often cover smaller employers than the ADA and also may cover a wider range of conditions. If you find yourself dealing with a potential pregnancy-related disability, consult your local civil rights agency or an attorney and see whether you might be entitled to accommodations on the job.

Our partners at WorkLife Law have prepared this sample doctor's notes for women who suffer from pregnancy-related impairments and seek coverage under the ADA. Be sure to read further in this section to learn more about doctor's notes and important caveats.

MEDICAL CERTIFICATION TO SUPPORT REQUEST FOR WORKPLACE ACCOMMODATION

PATIENT/EMPLOYEE/APPLICANT NAME: ___________

ADDRESS: ___________

EMPLOYER NAME: ___________

EMPLOYER ADDRESS: ___________

Dear Sir or Madam:

On June 15, 2014, my patient Ms. Jane Doe consulted with me in my office. I diagnosed Ms. Doe, who is pregnant, with carpal tunnel syndrome. Consistent with this diagnosis, Ms. Doe needs an accommodation at work until her baby is born, on or around November 1, 2014.

Because of Ms. Doe's carpal tunnel syndrome, and her associated limitation on repetitive use of both hands for more than 30 minutes without a break, she is having difficulty typing for long periods of time and should be allowed to take a 5-minute break after 30 minutes of continuous typing.

For more information, you may wish to consult the Job Accommodation Network at www.askjan.org.

NAME OF HEALTH CARE PROFESSIONAL: ___________

TYPE OF PRACTICE/MEDICAL SPECIALTY: ___________

ADDRESS: ___________

PHONE NUMBER / EMAIL: ___________

SIGNATURE / DATE: ___________

Workplace Accommodations for Healthy Pregnancies with Limitations

Even if your pregnancy is not complicated by any particular health concerns, you may find yourself unable to do certain parts of your job the way you used to or you may not want to do your regular work if it poses a risk to your or your baby's health. According to a recent survey,[13] a majority of women need some sort of change at work due to their pregnancy—more frequent breaks, such as bathroom breaks, are the most common request. A little over half of the women surveyed needed a change to job duties, like more sitting or less lifting. Unfortunately, a lot of women who needed accommodations did not ask for them (likely because of fear of retaliation), and others who did ask had their requests denied. Hopefully your employer will be understanding and willing to help you find a way to work around your limitations. Unfortunately, not all employers are so kind. Here are two true stories we heard in New York, the first from a physician and the second from one of our clinic callers:

> **In the spring of 2012, I treated a pregnant woman who arrived in the emergency department during my shift. She was working as a cashier at a large retailer in the city and was 16 weeks pregnant. Despite doctor's orders that she remain vigilant about drinking water, she was severely dehydrated. When I inquired why she was not drinking adequate amounts of fluids, she told me that her boss would not allow her to drink water while working at the cash register. While standing for hours at the register, the woman fainted and collapsed. She was rushed to the hospital by ambulance, where I ordered her intravenous fluids.**

A doctor's note changed the course of my life. When I pulled a muscle at six months pregnant, my doctor advised that I temporarily avoid heavy lifting while working for an armored truck company on Long Island. My boss took one look at the note and sent me home without pay indefinitely; the result was devastating. At six months pregnant, no one was willing to hire me. I had a four-year-old at home and was the primary income earner for our family. We fell behind in rent and applied for public assistance. Two weeks before my due date, I lost my health insurance. We struggled to put food on the table; it was an extremely difficult time.

These stories probably would not have happened in California,[14] where pregnant women are eligible for reasonable accommodations on the job even if their pregnancies are not disabling according to the law. If you are fortunate enough to work in California (a theme we'll return to *a lot*), you can take advantage of a specific law that requires employers to provide a reasonable accommodation for conditions related to pregnancy, childbirth, or related medical conditions, if an employee requests such an accommodation with the advice of her health care provider. Let's go back to the example of the cashier at the big-box store. Let's assume that she doesn't have gestational diabetes but does need to urinate frequently and can't comfortably stand on her feet for hours at a time. She has been advised by her doctor to sit while at work and to take more frequent breaks. Thanks to the law in California, the cashier can ask for—and probably receive—a stool and more bathroom breaks. These minimal changes to her schedule and workstation will allow her to take care of herself and her baby's health while also earning critical income her family needs.

And her employer keeps his employee on the job, avoiding the turnover costs of hiring and training a replacement. A win-win!

What types of accommodations might you request? Here's a list of some possible workplace changes that you might ask for to help you maintain a healthy pregnancy while working:

— Ability to sit for periods of time while on a shift
— Bathroom breaks
— Food or drink breaks
— Ability to carry water with you during work hours
— Flexibility around dress-code requirements
— Limits on lifting requirements
— Transfer to a less strenuous or hazardous shift, position, or work location
— Avoiding certain hazardous duties or chemicals, toxins, etc.
— Limited time off or altered work schedule to accommodate medical visits
— Reduced or flexible schedule

What if you are healthy and don't live in a state that provides better protections, such as California or New Jersey, but you still need a change at work—such as a bigger uniform? If your employer makes changes for other workers then they have to treat you the same (a common theme for this chapter). For example, if someone with a broken foot is allowed to alter the dress code, then you should be able to as well. Talk to your boss about your options: maybe you can wear maternity pants that are the same color as your uniform, even if they aren't an exact match, for example. Additionally, the fact that an employer refused to accommodate your pregnancy could suggest pregnancy discrimination, depend-

SAFETY FIRST

Are you shocked to hear there aren't more protections to ensure pregnant women's health and safety? Yet again, the United States is behind the times in comparison to other countries such as the United Kingdom and the countries of the European Union. In the United Kingdom, for example, employers have to assess the workplace to identify any risks to pregnant and breast-feeding women. And then the employer has to remove the risk or offer the mother alternate employment—or provide her with paid leave if neither option is possible.

ing on the circumstances. Talk to a lawyer to find out and look at our checklist at the end of this chapter to be sure you have covered all your bases.

Spotlight on NYC

New York City now has a law ensuring that pregnant workers in the city will not be pushed off the job when they need a modest accommodation in order to stay healthy and at work. Employers with four or more employees must provide reasonable accommodations for workers who have needs related to pregnancy or childbirth, or any pregnancy-related medical conditions. Employers have to comply with these requests, unless it would be an undue hardship—meaning, basically, that it would be really expensive or difficult. This means, for example, that a cashier at a Brooklyn pizza shop who is seven months pregnant and starting to get swollen feet from standing all day can request and receive a stool to sit on in front of the cash register or some other accommodation to let her keep working. For those of you working in NYC, here's a sample letter you could write to your employer if he or she denies your initial request for accommodation. Other workers in other jurisdictions that have similar laws (such as New Jersey) can use this as a template and adapt it.

SAMPLE LETTER TO YOUR SUPERVISOR IN NEW YORK CITY

TO: ____________________

FROM: ____________________

RE: The New York City Pregnant Workers Fairness Act

First, I want to thank you for your support during my [number] years with [company]. This is an exciting time for my family as we prepare for the birth of our child. I am eager to work with you to find a solution that will ensure I am able to be healthy and productive throughout my pregnancy.

As we discussed, I am requesting a reasonable accommodation so that I can continue working safely throughout my pregnancy. The New York City Pregnant Workers Fairness Act (PWFA) requires employers to provide reasonable accommodations to employees who have needs related to pregnancy, childbirth, and related medical conditions. I am entitled to this accommodation under the PWFA because I have a need related to my pregnancy, [company] has four or more employees, and because my requested accommodation would not cause an undue hardship on [company]. I know that additional local, state, and federal laws may also apply to my situation, such as the Pregnancy Discrimination

Act or the Americans with Disabilities Act Amendments Act.

According to a Job Accommodation Network (JAN) survey of over one thousand employers, the business benefits of providing reasonable accommodations to workers with disabilities far outweigh any cost. According to the survey, "Employers reported that providing accommodations resulted in such benefits as retaining valuable employees, improving productivity and morale, reducing workers' compensation and training costs, and improving company diversity." Since any needed accommodation associated with pregnancy is only short-term, the benefits of a policy of accommodating workers who are pregnant or recovering from childbirth are likely to be even greater and the costs even lower than those studied by JAN.

I look forward to working with you.

Sincerely,

[Your name]

Just What the Doctor Ordered

What if your employer asks you for a note from your medical provider verifying pregnancy limitations or specifying what you can and cannot do on the job? *Our advice: tread carefully*. Unfortunately, we have seen doctor's notes come back to bite employees all too often. Here's one example from one of our clinic callers:

I worked in a supermarket in New York City for eleven years. When I first became pregnant in 2005, I didn't ask for any accommodations because I was scared I would lose my job. I did heavy lifting and was worried the whole time about my health and my baby's health. Thankfully, I had a healthy pregnancy and gave birth to my first daughter. When I returned to my job from my

maternity leave my boss changed my shift to 5:30 a.m. in the morning, hoping I would quit. Waking up for a 5:30 am shift with a new baby was incredibly difficult, but I did it for two months until he finally changed my shift back. The next time I got pregnant in 2007 I told my manager and asked not to do any heavy lifting. He actually responded by giving me more heavy lifting to do. I think he was hoping I would quit. Sadly, I miscarried and suffered a series of miscarriages before finding out I had a blood clotting disorder.

After learning about this problem, the next time I got pregnant in 2009 I turned in a doctor's note to my boss with a five pound lifting restriction. The note also said I should take breaks when I was tired and shouldn't constantly go up and down stairs. My employer told me they had no job for me with those limitations, but I know they could have found work for me to do, like working in the deli. Another coworker had a shoulder problem and they accommodated her. They fired me, but thankfully my union helped me get disability payments for twenty-six weeks. Unfortunately, they were only a fraction of my usual salary. After the twenty-six weeks was up I had to go on unpaid leave for four months. I lost my health insurance and had to go on Medicaid. My family and I survived on food stamps and my savings. When I finally returned to work, I had nothing left in my savings account.

Many women believe that a note from their medical provider will protect them at work, and they feel more confident asking for a workplace modification with the support of such a note, but we have seen employers use medical notes to exclude women from their jobs altogether. We thought it would be best to go through some frequently asked questions here so you know what to expect if you find yourself needing a note from your provider. You should also take a look at our summary of "Talking to Your Boss About Your Bump" at the end of this chapter.

I need some changes at work because of a pregnancy-related condition. What if my employer says I have to get a note to continue working?

Sit down with your boss, and tell her that you have a pregnancy-related medical condition or need and require a "reasonable accommodation" (use that phrase). Come prepared with a plan—how do you propose to make this work? Ask for something reasonable, cheap, and relatively easy for your boss to provide that will allow you to continue performing the essential functions of your job. If she says no, then negotiate and ask what she would be willing to offer. Verify the conversation in writing afterward and take notes about your boss's reaction or anything she says during the meeting.

If your boss asks for a doctor's note verifying your request, try simply to put your request in writing and see if that is sufficient. If your boss still insists on a doctor's note, make sure your note is as specific as possible to address your pregnancy-related condition.

I am pregnant but don't need any changes to my work at this time. What if my employer still requires a doctor's note to allow me to keep working?

Unless your employer regularly requires employees who have disclosed medical conditions to provide doctors' notes to continue working, this kind of request may reveal a discriminatory motivation. Try putting in writing that you can and want to continue working as normal. Find out if others with medical conditions must bring in notes when they don't have any need for accommodations. If not, your employer can't single you out just because you are pregnant. Talk to your medical provider and find out if she would be willing to write a note that simply states that you have no pregnancy-related conditions or limitations and are capable of performing all essential functions of your job. If your employer has a general policy requiring employees have "no restrictions" to work, that is most likely a violation of disability laws.

I decided I want to bring in a doctor's note—is there anything it should say or should not say?

First, take a look at the state-by-state guide and talk with your provider to find out if you have any problems related to your pregnancy that may qualify for coverage under disability law. If so, then take a look at the sample doctor's notes for disabilities earlier in this chapter. If not, then we recommend using the sample note from California (see below) for guidance. The most important thing to remember is that the requested accommodation and described restrictions should be as specific as possible. For example, your doctor should avoid general prescriptions like you "need light duty" or "should minimize heavy lifting." These recommendations are too vague and will only lead to problems at work—you might even be pushed out of the workplace indefinitely, or until your employer has clarification. Similarly, notes that say you cannot lift more than fifteen to twenty pounds should be more specific. Does this mean you can't lift more than fifteen pounds or more than twenty pounds, or does it depend on some other factor? Can you lift that much sometimes or never? What if you get assistance? Ask your doctor to tailor the letter to the duties at work that you need to avoid. For example, if you never lift heavy things, but do push heavy carts or patients, have the note specify how much weight you can push, not how much weight you can lift (you can push a lot more weight on wheels than you can lift!).

Help! I'm being pushed out even though I want to keep working. What now?

Ask a lot of questions and assert that you want to keep working and can keep working. Let them do the talking and then take careful notes afterward. The more you listen and ask questions, the more you will understand their motivations, which could very well be illegal. You may suspect pregnancy discrimination, but it's better to have proof—like an email from your boss making stereotypical assumptions about your work because of your pregnancy. Here are some things to watch out for and take note of:

— Any concerns your employer expresses about your health or the fetus's health.
— Any concerns your employer mentions about her own liability.
— Offensive comments about your pregnancy or family.
— Did your employer ask for a doctor's note before you even requested any accommodations?
— Do others have to get a doctor's note, like someone who needs an accommodation for a disability or injury?
— Does your employer have any policies (either in writing or that she has told you about) that effectively exclude pregnant women from the workplace (like an unrealistic requirement to lift fifty pounds)?

Talk to a lawyer and be sure to mention any of the above that you have observed. They could be evidence of pregnancy discrimination. Even if your employer seems like she is looking out for you—maybe she says she doesn't want your baby to be hurt—that could still be illegal. Courts have long recognized that paternalistic concerns for pregnant women's health have been used to limit women's rights.

My employer says they don't have "light duty," but I can't do heavy lifting like I did before I was pregnant, what should I do?

Gather information to make a case for yourself—does your employer provide light duty for other workers, like those who are injured on-the-job or those who are disabled? Most, but not all, employers do. If so, then you may be entitled to light duty under the Pregnancy Discrimination Act. Is there a light duty position available that you could fill? Could you simply shift some of your duties to a coworker, or do you need a temporary transfer to another position? Try to work it out with your employer and explain that any changes are only temporary. If your employer requires a doctor's note, be sure to check if you have a problem that may qualify you for coverage under disability law (see page 183) and be sure that the doctor's note is very specific (outlining exactly how much weight you can lift and how often). If your employer truly doesn't provide light duty to anyone else and there are no other options, at least try to get your boss to hold your job open for you so you can return after giving birth.

I live in California, do I have to give my employer a doctor's note?

Yes, the law does require that you request an accommodation based upon the advice of your health care provider. Our partners at the Legal Aid Society—Employment Law Center, based in San Francisco, have prepared this sample doctor's note for California women requesting a reasonable accommodation:

Your Health Care
Provider's Letterhead

[Date]

To Whom It May Concern:

I am the [treating physician, nurse practitioner, nurse midwife, licensed midwife, clinical psychologist, clinical social worker, licensed marriage or family therapist, licensed acupuncturist, physician assistant, chiropractor, social worker, or health care professional] for [Your Name].

[Name] has a condition related to [pregnancy or childbirth]. [Note: This can be any physical or mental condition that is intrinsic to pregnancy or childbirth, including, but not limited to, lactation. You do NOT need to reveal a diagnosis or details of the condition, but you do need to state that the patient has a condition related to pregnancy or childbirth.]

As a result of [Name]'s condition, it is medically advisable that she receive the following accommodation: [Describe requested accommodation here. E.g., to avoid lifting over [X] lbs., to avoid climbing ladders, to avoid exposure to toxic fumes, permission to drink water or snack during her shift, a larger uniform, a modified work schedule, more frequent bathroom breaks, a stool or chair to sit on, additional break time and a private space to express breast milk, a temporary transfer to a less strenuous or hazardous position].

This accommodation became medically advisable on [Date]. At this time, I anticipate that [Name] will need this accommodation for [duration of accommodation].

Thank you.

[Signature]

My employer wants to talk to my doctor directly—should I allow that?

We think it's best if you stay involved in any conversations between your medical provider and your employer. Your provider needs your permission to say anything to your employer about your medical condition, so you should be clear when giving that permission that you want to be present for any and all conversations. This way you can stick up for yourself if you need to, but you will also know exactly what was said in any meetings.

My employer has a form she wants my doctor to fill out so I can keep working—it's a checklist saying what I can and cannot do at work. Does my doctor need to fill this out?

It's best if your provider can explain in his or her own words what limitations or restrictions you may have. Unfortunately, checklists can lead to confusion or miscommunication. First, see if a note from your provider can replace the checklist. If that won't fly, then have your provider fill out the checklist, but include an accompanying letter to provide explanation and clarification. The provider can then attach a note. As we have discussed, be prepared that checking off that you cannot perform a particular task may be used to push you out of the workplace.

I have a doctor's appointment tomorrow, what should I ask my doctor?

It's important to talk to your medical provider about your job duties before you announce that you are pregnant at work. Make a list of the functions you do on a typical day and the things you do infrequently. Take a look at your job description (from the handbook or when you were hired), this can help you make a list of not only what you do, but also what your employer says you need to be ready to do at work. Write down any chemicals, toxins, or other hazards (like radiation), that you may have exposure to. Be sure to write down, before your appointment, any concerns or questions you have about your work.

Go through each item with your provider to find out if there's anything you need to worry about, either at this stage or later as your pregnancy progresses. Of course, some women who have been pregnant before or who feel comfortable with their job duties may not need to do this, but for those who have questions, it's best to come prepared since medical providers may not understand what kind of work different jobs entail. A retail worker may be exposed to harmful cleaning chemicals, for example, if she needs to clean up the store, but a doctor may not realize that unless the patient brings it to his attention.

Checklist for Staying Healthy and On the Job While Pregnant

1. Check your employer's policies to see whether you are entitled to accommodations while pregnant. If you are a union member, check your Collective Bargaining Agreement and speak with your Union Representative or Shop Steward.
2. Talk to your doctor to find out if you have any diseases, disorders, illnesses, or other medical problems to see if you might qualify for coverage under disability law, as discussed earlier in this chapter. Even if you don't think of yourself as "disabled," you could be covered, especially by more expansive state and local laws, if, for example, you have pelvic pain or shortness of breath. If you are found to have some form of a disability, then disability laws may entitle you to a reasonable accommodation.

3. Check to see if your state or city has a law that guarantees the right to seek accommodations for your pregnancy.
4. Check your employer's policies about others with limitations at work, such as those with disabilities or on-the-job injuries and ask around to find out how others temporarily unable to do some job duties have been treated by your employer.

If the rest of your checklist came up empty, and your employer is not required by law to help you, then try appealing to your boss's humanity and to her bottom line or seeing if coworkers might be able to cover some of your duties. You may also want to talk to an attorney to find out if your employer's policy or the fact that she refused to accommodate you may be evidence of pregnancy or disability discrimination.

SICK AND TIRED: TIME OFF FOR PREGNANCY-RELATED ILLNESS AND PRENATAL CARE

My first pregnancy was horrible in the beginning. I suffered from hyperemesis, when your body cannot tolerate the pregnancy hormones and you are so sick that you lose weight instead of gaining it. I didn't dare say anything to my employer because I knew that they did not care about anything but my billable hours. In fact, I was terrified to tell them I was pregnant because I thought they would discriminate against me. So I suffered through it.

As many expecting parents know, "morning sickness" is not always limited to the early hours of the day. In fact, nausea, fatigue, headaches, and more can dog a pregnant woman all day and for months at a stretch. It can be hard to keep up with work when you are struggling to stay upright or keep food down. Many pregnant women recover their energy in the second trimester, but for some the sickness persists throughout the whole pregnancy. And on top of all that, a good number of pregnant women need to go on bed rest toward the end of their pregnancies, to avoid preterm delivery. So what should you do if your pregnancy forces you to miss work?

The law protects you in several ways. First of all, the Pregnancy Discrimination Act (PDA) requires that your employer treat you the same as any coworker who also has to miss work because he or she is similarly unable to work. So if a colleague has to miss work periodically over a few months for medical treatment or for continuing education classes, and your employer allows him or her to do so without penalty, the same rule should apply to you. Or imagine one of your colleagues injures his knee playing basketball and has to keep his leg elevated for a few weeks. If your employer allows the coworker to work from home while his knee recovers, he or she should also allow you to work from home while you are on bed rest. Similarly, if your employer provides paid sick time, he or she has to allow you to use that time for your pregnancy-related illness and absences.

Second, if you are eligible for leave under the Family and Medical Leave Act (FMLA, which we discuss in much greater detail in chapter 2), you are entitled to time off for pregnancy-related illness, bed rest, and prenatal appointments. The law is more lenient in the case of pregnancy than for other disabling conditions: you don't have to be under the care of a doctor or be absent for more than three days to qualify for this kind of time off. So let's say you are late to work one day because you spent the morning face to face with your toilet bowl; you can count that time as FMLA leave (see chapter 2 for more information). Even if you are late by only a few minutes, you may be able to count this time off as protected leave. This is called "intermittent leave" in the law. One downside is that any FMLA time you take before your baby is born is time you won't have for bonding leave after he or she arrives—you get only up to twelve weeks in a twelve-month period, and all FMLA-qualifying time you take in that twelve-month period counts toward your total.

Samantha worked for nearly two years as a receptionist at a large nonprofit. At thirty-two weeks into her pregnancy, she was struggling with health problems related to her pregnancy and was coming in late and missing work a lot as a result. Unfortunately, Samantha had already used up her sick leave, and her boss said that he wanted her to start her maternity leave early, after first taking five days of her accrued vacation leave. Samantha did not want to start maternity leave early, preferring to work further into her pregnancy, even though she knew there would be times when she would have to call in sick. Samantha's employer was supposed to grant her FMLA leave intermittently, which would allow her to stay on the job and use unpaid time off for her doctor visits. She could still use the bulk of her leave after her baby arrived, rather than losing the last few months of pay. Instead, Samantha's employer forced her out on disability, and the insurance company denied her claim for benefits. Samantha's employer expected her to return to work within a matter of weeks after giving birth, but she

TIME-OUT FOR OUTRAGE!

Our allies across the Atlantic do far more for their mums-to-be. All pregnant employees in the United Kingdom, no matter how long they have been working in their jobs, are entitled to reasonable time off from work for prenatal care. This time may include childbirth and parenting classes as well as medical examinations—and pregnant workers must be paid at their regular rate of pay for this time off! Compare this to the FMLA, which covers only half the private-sector workforce, guarantees only unpaid time off, and guarantees leave only for those pregnant women who have worked for at least a year for their employer. On top of that, any FMLA time taken for prenatal care is time you won't have for maternity leave. Meanwhile, new moms in the United Kingdom have one whole year of maternity leave, the majority of which is paid, and are eligible for that leave no matter how long they have worked for their employer or how many hours they work.

Are you outraged yet? And we're not even talking about Sweden!

To read more about the United Kingdom's policies on their extremely accessible and user-friendly website, visit www.direct.gov.uk and navigate to "Employment" and then "Work and Families" ("Parents" section).

could not afford the only day care program that would accept her infant son. Samantha ultimately lost her job and her primary source of income.

Although the law can help you manage the challenges of pregnancy-related illness at work, there are limits. Like we said previously, the law just requires employers to treat pregnant women the same way they treat everybody else. Unless you are eligible for FMLA leave or disability law coverage, your employer is not required to provide you with any time off to deal with pregnancy-related sickness or medical visits if it does not provide time off for other employees' illnesses or medical treatment. In other words, if your workplace does not provide any leave for any employees, your employer doesn't have to make an exception for you, under federal law, just because you are pregnant. This is, unfortunately, the harsh reality of the law. Employers can treat everyone poorly, and it's perfectly legal. In some cases, lawyers have tried to prove that such a severe policy, although neutral on its face, has an illegal negative impact on women because of their ability to become pregnant. In fact, the Equal Opportunity Employment Commission—the federal agency in charge of enforcing employment discrimination laws—says that if a pregnant worker is fired because her employer doesn't offer enough, or any, leave that may be discriminatory if the policy is not justified by business necessity and if it disproportionately harms women.[15]

Although there are multiple ways to prove discrimination, the PDA may often involve comparison between a pregnant woman and a nonpregnant coworker to determine whether an employer is being fair. What if there is no other worker at your workplace who is similar to you in his or her inability to work? In one real case, Ms. Troupe, a pregnant saleswoman at a department store, suffered from chronic and debilitating morning sickness, and was fired for excessive tardiness. She brought a lawsuit alleging discrimination but lost. The court said she needed to prove that the store would have fired a "hypothetical Mr. Troupe" with a similar record of tardiness and plans for medical leave. But proving such an unknown can be almost impossible, not to mention costly and time-consuming. And discrimination lawsuits can take years to play out, delaying any resolution until long past your due date. (Note that the FMLA *might* require an employer to give some time off in this kind of case, as we discuss more in chapter 2.)

As we discuss throughout the book, when it looks like federal law leaves you high and dry, always check to see whether you are entitled to any additional time off or protections under your state or local law. For example, in San Francisco, Seattle, Washington, DC, Portland, New York City, in the state of Connecticut, and several other localities, many employees are guaranteed paid sick time by law, which they may use for pregnancy-related illness and medical care. Or as we discussed earlier in this chapter, you may be entitled to some kind of accommodation or modification of your schedule because of your pregnancy or pregnancy-related illness.

Checklist for Sick Leave

1. Check your employer's policies to see what time off you may be allowed in the form of sick leave, personal time, or paid time off. If you are entitled to sick time, you must be able to use that time for prenatal appointments or morning sickness under the law. If you are a union member, check

your Collective Bargaining Agreement and speak with your Union Representative or Shop Steward.

2. Check to see whether you are eligible for time off under the Family and Medical Leave Act (see chapter 2 for more details). You may be able to use this time for complications and illness related to pregnancy so that you can keep working further into your pregnancy.
3. Check to see what, if anything, may be guaranteed to you by state or local laws, in terms of time off for your pregnancy or pregnancy-related illness, such as paid sick days laws or disability laws.
4. Check your employer's policies about temporary disabilities and ask around to find out how others temporarily unable to work have been treated by your employer.

If the rest of your checklist came up empty, and your employer is not required by law to help you, try appealing to your boss's humanity and to his or her bottom line or seeing if coworkers might be able to cover your shift while you are out.

Talking to Your Boss About Your Bump

This fact sheet focuses on federal law. Your state or local laws may provide different/broader protections.

WHEN to break the news:

- There are no real legal deadlines for notifying your employer until late in your pregnancy, when you will need to request leave thirty days in advance of taking off for childbirth, if you are covered by the Family and Medical Leave Act.

- If you need time off for pregnancy-related illness, or you need another workplace change to accommodate your pregnancy, you may have to break the news earlier.
- If you suspect that your boss won't be happy to hear you are pregnant, don't feel pressure to tell before you are ready. However, keep in mind that your colleagues and boss may appreciate being told as soon as you feel comfortable, so that they, and you, can plan ahead.

WHAT *to say*:

- Before starting the conversation, it's a good idea to do your homework and review your employer's policies about pregnancy and parental leave. You may also want to consult with human resources.
- Reassure your boss that *you are committed to your job* and that you plan to return to work after the baby arrives. Many bosses wrongly assume that pregnancy means the end of an employee's dedication and reliability. It's important to tackle those assumptions up front.
- Stress that *you are willing and able to keep working*—even if your pregnancy impacts your work, it will be a short-term situation, like a temporary disability. You don't need a doctor's note to announce your pregnancy, and in fact, sometimes a note can cause trouble if your boss thinks it limits what you can do on the job.
- Highlight that you are a breadwinner (or primary earner) for your family, and your household depends on your paycheck.
- If you have access to parental leave, *come armed with a plan to help your boss prepare for your absence* and cover your workload while you are gone.
- Listen carefully and take careful notes after your conversation, especially about anything that sounded strange or wrong to you.

- Unfair treatment based on pregnancy (e.g. firing or penalizing you upon learning you are pregnant) is illegal.
- Depending on your situation and the city or state you work in, you may have a right to workplace changes to accommodate your pregnancy.

Workplace Accommodations

Have a conversation with your medical provider about your job duties to understand if you may need changes at work because of your pregnancy, such as time off for prenatal appointments or nausea, a stool to sit on, the ability to carry a water bottle, a change to your uniform, limiting heavy lifting, frequent bathroom breaks, or anything else. Keep in mind that your needs may change over the course of your pregnancy. If you do want to seek an accommodation, keep reading!

HOW to ask for an accommodation:

FIRST: If you work in California, Hawaii, Louisiana, Connecticut, Maryland, Iowa, New Jersey, West Virginia, Minnesota, Texas, Illinois, Alaska, New York City, Philadelphia, or Central Falls, Rhode Island, state or local law may guarantee you the right to certain workplace modifications. Check with your local civil rights agency or visit www.abetterbalance.org to find out more and remember that the advice below may differ a bit if you live in one of the places listed above.

SECOND: Do you have a diagnosed medical condition or disability associated with your pregnancy, like gestational diabetes, hypertension, migraines, fatigue, back pain, or swelling in your feet? If so, federal and/or state disability law should protect you.

- Tell your boss that you have a *disability or complication arising from your pregnancy* and that you *need a reasonable accommodation* on the job. Look at the list on pg. 186 of pregnancy-related conditions and possible workplace accommodations.

- *Specify* what kind of accommodation you need, including any job duties that you need modified, and make sure your boss knows you can still *perform the bulk of the duties of your job*. Refer your boss to the Job Accommodation Network (http://askjan.org/soar/other/preg.html) for more information and ideas.
- *Come prepared with a plan*–what kind of changes do you need and how can you make that work? Talk with coworkers and enlist their help.
- Explain how your requested accommodation *will not be too difficult or expensive for the company* (e.g. it's time limited, another employee is willing to help you on occasion with the task you can't perform, etc.)
- This should be a two-way conversation–your boss must engage with you. If she asks for additional information, you should provide it. Make sure to get the conversation documented in writing–you may send an email or note summing up what was discussed and keep a copy for your records.

THIRD: If you *don't* have any complications or disabilities related to your pregnancy and simply need to ensure you can continue working comfortably and maintain a healthy pregnancy:

- Tell your boss you *need a reasonable accommodation for your pregnancy* so that you can continue to do your job safely.
- *Come prepared with a plan*–what kind of changes do you need and how can you make that work? Talk with coworkers and enlist their help.
- Explain that the changes you seek are small and will *not impose an undue hardship* on the company (i.e. not too costly or difficult).

- Keep in mind that if your employer accommodates workers with disabilities, and those with on-the-job injuries, *under the Pregnancy Discrimination Act they should do the same for you.*
- If you are eligible, you may use time under the Family and Medical Leave Act for prenatal checkups and smaller chunks of time when your pregnancy makes it impossible for you to report to work. Give your employer advance notice (thirty days if possible) for time off related to your pregnancy.

FOURTH: If your boss requires a note from your doctor to confirm your medical need, *make sure that the doctor's note is as specific as possible* and outlines exactly what you can and cannot do at work. *Avoid vague terms like "heavy lifting" or "light duty,"* which may be interpreted by your boss to mean you can no longer do your job. Be aware that employers often use doctor's notes to say that pregnant women can't do their jobs and to push them out of the workplace, either by forcing them onto leave before they are ready or by firing them outright.

Hopefully, we've been able to answer a lot of your questions about how to handle the legal issues that may pop up during the first nine months of your journey into parenthood. We've included a resource list for this chapter later in the book, if you want to continue your research. Now you are ready for the next phase—bonding with baby, the subject of our next chapter.

TOP FIVE THINGS TO REMEMBER

- You may be entitled to some workplace modifications if you suffer from pregnancy complications or if your employer offers modifications to other workers.
- You cannot be forced out onto leave or out of your job just because you are pregnant, as long as you can do the work.
- You don't necessarily have to be pregnant at the time you experience discrimination to be protected by the law.
- Employers can't refuse to hire you just because you are, or may become, pregnant.
- State laws may offer more protections for you, so be sure to do your homework!

2 TIME TO BOND
Planning for Parental Leave

• POP QUIZ •

True or False?

1. **Everybody in the United States gets at least twelve weeks off work when they have a new baby.**
   False. Only about half the private workforce is entitled to leave of that length.

2. **But that's okay because most employers provide paid maternity leave anyway.**
   False. Only about 16 percent of private employers offer paid maternity leave.

3. **Depending on which state you live in, you could get as much as $1,000 per week in leave benefits–or nothing.**
   True. Location, location, location.

Nine months of pregnancy can feel like an eternity, and the adoption process can drag on even longer. But someday the waiting *will* end, and you will officially become a parent. Nothing can really prepare you for the sweeping emotions and sleepless nights of early parenthood. But if you can increase your time with your baby and reduce your stress in those early days, you will improve your odds for success. Planning ahead is key.

So what are you entitled to for maternity/parental leave? There is no simple answer. Your rights will depend on where you live and where you work. As we mentioned earlier, maternity leave varies tremendously from country to country, but it also varies from one state to the next (take a look at the end of this chapter—How the Other Half Lives: Leave Options beyond the FMLA—for an example!). If you work for state or federal government, you likely will have different rights than your private-sector friends. If you are in a union, you may be entitled to more time off than nonunionized workers. If you work for a large employer, you'll probably benefit from more time off than new parents who work for a small enterprise. And if you are a birth mother, you may be entitled to more time off than your partner. That's a lot of "ifs"! Where do you start?

In this chapter, we review the federal and state laws that may entitle you to some time off work to recover from childbirth or to bond with your new baby. It's important to remember that there are two different types of leave (pregnancy/disability leave vs. bonding leave) that may be covered by different laws. We start with the Family and Medical Leave Act, which is the one federal law designed to give new parents time off to bond with their babies. Then we review state laws that may guarantee you leave time or some wage replacement (i.e., money!) for the time you are disabled from childbirth or pregnancy or (in three states) for time you spend bonding with your new child or caring for a pregnant partner. We also discuss where else to look for help and how to plan ahead if the law does not cover you or your employer.

FAMILY AND MEDICAL LEAVE ACT OF 1993

"Fim-La," "FMLA," "Family Leave"—have you heard these terms in passing but not known what folks were talking about? These are common nicknames for the Family and Medical Leave Act of 1993 (FMLA), which is the one parental leave law that applies across the country to workers in every state. This complicated law basically lets some employees take time away from work in order to care for themselves or family members. It guarantees time off for pregnancy-related illness, for prenatal medical visits, and for recovery from childbirth. It provides time off for bonding with a newborn or newly adopted child and also guarantees workers time to care for themselves or an immediate family member who is seriously ill.

Sounds great, right? Before you get too excited, you should know that your employer is not required to pay you while you are out on FMLA leave. And we must warn you that the FMLA is limited in its reach. In fact, the law covers only about half of the private-sector workforce in the United States. And it is pretty complex to boot. So before you travel with us into the FMLA's murky depths, make sure it applies to you. For starters, you can check out our handy nutshell below and read the section of this chapter on eligibility. If you have any doubts, you should speak with an attorney. And keep in mind, even if the law does not apply to you or your employer now, it may apply to your partner or to you in the future. Information is power, so if you have the patience (and time), stick with us and learn more!

The FMLA in a Nutshell

WHAT?

- Up to twelve weeks of unpaid leave for pregnant moms or new parents to care for their own serious health condition and/or to bond with a new child within one year of birth or adoption. Leave is also available to care for a seriously ill immediate family member.
- Leave may be taken intermittently–that is, not all at once but in smaller bits. Employers must approve of intermittent leave in the case of bonding leave.
- Leave-takers are guaranteed continued benefits such as health insurance while on leave and are guaranteed their job back, or an equivalent one, upon return to work, unless they are in the top 10 percent of the company (measured by salary).
- Employers may not interfere with or retaliate against an employee for exercising his or her rights under the law.

WHERE?

All government employers and those private employers with fifty or more employees within a seventy-five-mile radius of each other must comply with the law.

WHO?

Employees who have worked for a covered employer for at least twelve months and have worked at least 1,250 hours in the twelve months before taking leave.

WHEN?

Eligible employees may take up to twelve weeks of leave within a twelve-month period that is determined by the employer.

HOW?

Employees who know about their need for leave in advance must give their employer at least thirty days of notice. If leave is unpredictable, they must give notice as soon as practicable. Employees must also give enough information for the employer to understand that they are seeking FMLA-covered time off.

ARE YOU IN OR OUT?
WHO IS COVERED UNDER THE FMLA?

How do I know whether I can take FMLA leave?

About half of all workers cannot take FMLA leave at all because they work for an employer that is not big enough or because they do not personally qualify.

In order to be eligible for FMLA leave, you must work for an employer that is covered by the law *and* you must qualify for leave.

Covered employers include:

— any private-sector employer who employs fifty or more people (each day during each of twenty or more calendar workweeks in the current or preceding year)

— any state, local, or federal government agency, no matter how many people it employs

— any public or private elementary or secondary school, regardless of the number of employees

Eligible employees include those who:

— are employed by one of the employers listed previously

— have been employed there for at least twelve months (although not necessarily twelve months in a row)
— worked at least 1,250 hours during the twelve months right before taking leave
— work at a location where they are within seventy-five miles of at least fifty other employees working for their employer

So, for example, if you work for an employer that has more than one hundred employees, but they are scattered throughout the country, and you work at a location with only ten others, and the next worksite is two states over, you may not be eligible for FMLA leave. However, if you have worked forty hours a week for a big corporation for two years, then you are probably able to benefit from the FMLA.

Why does the law include these complicated eligibility requirements?
They are part of a legislative compromise by our representatives in Washington. Many lawmakers were concerned that a family leave law would burden small businesses, so they made plenty of exceptions and carve-outs.

My employer never told me about my FMLA rights. Do they have to tell me about my leave options?
If your employer is covered by the FMLA, then yes. They have to post about the law conspicuously and put it in any employee handbooks or otherwise distribute it to any new employees.

What does my employer have to include in the notice?
The notice has to explain the FMLA's provisions and provide information about how to file a complaint. Also, once your boss

has reason to believe that you may need to take FMLA leave, she or he has to notify you of your eligibility within five business days. This means that even if you don't use the word "FMLA," but instead say something like "I'm having a baby," your employer has to let you know about the law, if you are eligible.

What if I work part-time?

You have to have worked at least 1,250 hours total in the twelve months before your first day of leave. This unfortunately excludes many people who work part-time. Employees who work forty hours per week work about 2,080 hours in a year (assuming they are working fifty-two full weeks in a year). Working 1,250 hours

ADOPTING A CHILD

If you are thinking about adopting a child, then you probably already know that adoption can require time for appointments even before a new child is welcomed into your home. If you adopt a child, you are entitled to twelve weeks of leave to bond with and care for the child within twelve months after placement in the same way as someone who gave birth to a child. Adoptive parents are also allowed to take FMLA leave prior to placement if they need to miss work in order to complete the adoption. You can miss work to attend counseling sessions, appear in court, consult with your attorney or the doctor representing the birth parent, submit to a physical examination, or travel to another country. The preceding list is not exhaustive.

comes out to working a little more than twenty-four hours per week, assuming fifty-two weeks in a year, or a little over 104 hours per month; it comes out to working twenty-five hours per week for fifty weeks exactly.

I work twenty-five hours per week, but I wasn't in the office for three weeks in the last year because I took a paid vacation. Do I qualify?

If you worked twenty-five hours per week for forty-nine weeks, then you worked only 1,225 hours, and you would not qualify. The FMLA does not count paid vacation or other paid days off; it counts only the days you were actually working.

I worked for my employer for three years and then went to school for two years. I came back to the same employer and have worked there now for eight months. I am pregnant and want to take FMLA leave when my baby arrives. Am I eligible?

Yes, as long as you worked 1,250 hours in the twelve months prior to the start of your leave. Although you must work at least twelve months for your employer to be eligible for leave, those months do not have to be all in a row. Your three years of work before you went to school will count toward your FMLA eligibility. If you took a break of seven years or more, however, your employer wouldn't have to count your earlier employment *unless* that break was due to military service or you had a written agreement that your employer would rehire you after your time away.

FMLA 101: The Basic Protections of the FMLA

What kind of leave does the FMLA provide?

Twelve workweeks of leave in a twelve-month period for the following circumstances:

— the birth of a child and care for the newborn child within one year of birth

— the placement with the employee of a child for adoption or foster care and care for the newly placed child within one year of placement

— care for the employee's spouse, child, or parent who has a serious health condition

— a serious health condition that makes the employee unable to perform the essential functions of his or her job

— any qualifying exigency arising out of the fact that the employee's spouse, son, daughter, or parent is a covered military member on "covered active duty"

— twenty-six workweeks of leave during a single twelve-month period to care for a covered service member with a serious injury or illness who is the spouse, son, daughter, parent, or next of kin to the employee (military caregiver leave).

Am I guaranteed my job back?

Yes, you are entitled to the same position or an equivalent position unless you are a "key employee," defined as the top 10 percent of employees based on salary.

For example, a corporation would be within its rights to terminate a CEO taking FMLA leave.

What does "the same or equivalent job" mean?
An equivalent position means equivalent benefits, pay, and other terms and conditions of employment. For example, shorter shifts and lower pay after returning to work is definitely *not* equal to the same job.

What qualifies as a "serious health condition" under the law?
This is a fairly broad term covering overnight stays in the hospital, conditions that make you or a loved one unable to work or go to school for more than three days. For example, taking time off for chemotherapy or taking time to treat serious asthma both would likely count. Upset stomachs and the common cold are not serious health conditions, however, unless complications arise. If you are incapacitated because of your pregnancy, you may take FMLA leave for that time, even if you are not under the care of a doctor and even if you are absent from work for only a day or two.

I took two paid sick days a few months ago when I had a stomach bug; can my employer deduct those two days from my twelve weeks of FMLA leave?
No, because you were not using the time off for an FMLA-qualifying reason, since the stomach bug was not a serious medical condition. Your employer also can't retroactively designate time you took off as FMLA-qualifying when you were up front about why you were out.

Can I use FMLA leave to cover my prenatal doctor appointments, doctor-ordered bed rest, and severe morning sickness? (And do I have to?)
Yes, you can definitely take FMLA leave for prenatal care. You can also take FMLA leave if your condition makes you unable to

work. This is the case even if you do not receive treatment from a doctor throughout the leave (which is required for other serious health conditions). You also need not be absent for more than three days (another requirement for other illnesses). Therefore, even if you are just a few minutes late due to severe morning sickness, you still may be able to count that time off as FMLA leave.

You might be thinking that you would rather use paid sick time for these absences so that you can save the full twelve weeks of FMLA leave for the weeks after your baby arrives. Some employers allow this, if an employee requests it. But unfortunately, your

Opting Out?

As we've said, one of the major problems with FMLA leave is that it is unpaid–in fact, a recent Department of Labor survey found that more than half of workers who were FMLA-eligible and did not take leave, cited lack of payment as the reason.[16] If workers can't afford to take leave to have children, then what do they do? A recent survey of college graduates reveals one answer: some are opting out of having children entirely. These graduates cite a number of factors, such as anticipated work/family conflict in their careers, longer work hours, and increased student loan debt. A generation-wide baby embargo can be dangerous for all of us. As our country's birthrate levels off, elected officials have additional economic, as well as moral, reasons to provide more robust work/family protections for all Americans.

employer can force you to use FMLA leave so that you are not out of work for longer than twelve weeks total if you are absent for an FMLA-qualifying reason. And keep in mind that if you use paid sick leave for doctor appointments but later decide to reveal to your employer that they were prenatal appointments, your employer may be able to go back and apply FMLA leave to the time you took for the appointments.

Will my doctor have to give my employer all my medical records if I request FMLA leave?

No, all your employer can get is a "medical certification," which is a form that contains only the facts needed to establish that you have a serious medical condition qualifying for FMLA leave (in your case, pregnancy). For example, that means your employer does not get to find out your HIV status or whether you previously had an abortion, because that is not needed to establish that you are pregnant. If you are seeking to keep your pregnancy itself under wraps, that could be trickier. For example, if you want to use FMLA leave for a prenatal appointment or nausea but do not yet want your employer to know you are pregnant, you might say, "I need to go to an appointment for an FMLA-qualifying reason" or "I have to come in late due to a medical condition that is covered by the FMLA." You do not have to produce a doctor's note to prove you are pregnant before taking intermittent FMLA leave for prenatal care or pregnancy-related sickness. However, if you do not announce your pregnancy, your employer may then request medical certification from a doctor, which may reveal your pregnancy.

Can my spouse and I both take FMLA leave to care for our new baby?

Yes. Both parents can take "bonding time" until their child's first birthday. For example, a mother could take twelve weeks off from work immediately after giving birth, and her partner could then take the following twelve weeks to care for the new child, allowing the baby twenty-four weeks total of exclusive parent care. The parents could also choose to take the twelve weeks together to bond with the baby as a family. However, if the couple works for the same employer, they may be limited to twelve weeks total between the two of them for bonding leave.

Daddy Duty

Fathers are allowed to take FMLA leave to care for their newborn children for twelve weeks, just like mothers. Unfortunately, many men don't take nearly that much time off, in part because of the stigma they feel if they prioritize family over work and because FMLA leave is unpaid. Here are some real quotes from dads we surveyed about this:

> **"I took a month of [partial] family leave for the birth of my son and this led to negative perception regarding my dedication. This was so even though I continued to work about thirty to thirty-five hours per week (a typical week was about sixty hours)."**
>
> **–finance professional and father of one child, age three**

"When I first asked for the time off, the CFO said, 'If we can do without someone for a whole month, I wonder if we need the position at all . . .'"

–nonprofit professional and father of one child, age three

"If I could have afforded it, it would have been nice to take a full three months off to help my wife when my sons were born."

–designer and father of infant triplets

"I was told I would be fired if I took off for my son's birth."

–information technology professional and father of one child, age two

Contrast these experiences with those of dads in Sweden, who get sixty days of *paid* parental leave reserved just for them!

Do I keep my benefits while on leave?

Your employer must maintain your health insurance coverage under any group health plans. However, if you inform your employer that you will not return to work after your leave period, they can immediately cut off your health insurance benefits. In some cases an employer may even be able to recover premiums paid during leave if you fail to return to work after FMLA leave. Even if you do return to work, if you then decide to quit within thirty days, your employer can reclaim from you all the money it spent on your health insurance premiums while you were out on leave.

Your employer has no obligation to provide other benefits, such as holiday pay, while you are on leave.

Do I have to pay my health insurance premiums while on leave?
If a portion of your premium is typically taken out of your paycheck, then you will need to work out an arrangement with your employer to continue paying your share of the premiums. Additionally, an employer is not obligated to pay the premiums anymore if the employee is very late with a premium payment (and a couple of other requirements are met).

How much contact should/must I have with work while I'm on leave?
Generally speaking, when you are on leave, you are not working, and your employer should respect that. You should not feel pressured to be in touch until discussion of your return date. Although your employer may reach out with update calls or emails, demanding real work product from you while on leave could be considered illegal interference with your rights under the FMLA. That being said, it's probably a good idea to keep in touch to some extent, so your employer knows you remain committed to your job. Before heading out on leave, let your employer know how you would like to communicate while you are out and designate a point of contact for anything urgent that may come up.

Someone to Watch Over Me: What If You Need Care?

Can my partner use his or her FMLA leave to care for me during my pregnancy?
Yes, if you are a heterosexual married couple or a same-sex married couple living in a state that respects your marriage. However, you cannot take FMLA leave to care for your same-sex spouse, even if you are legally married, if the state where you live does not recognize your marriage. This is because existing FMLA regulations define "spouse" based on the laws of the state in which an

employee *lives*, rather than the laws of the state where the marriage was performed. However this rule may change soon, so make sure to check with the US Department of Labor or A Better Balance if you are a married same-sex couple living in a state that does not recognize your marriage—you may be covered by the FMLA by the time you're reading this!

The FMLA does not cover domestic partnerships or civil unions.

The rules for federal employees are different. Federal employees who are legally married to a person of the same-sex can take FMLA leave to care for their same-sex spouses even if they live in a state that does not recognize their marriage. Contact A Better Balance if you face problems or have questions about your rights as an LGBT federal employee.

Finally, you may have additional rights to family and medical leave under state law. Check out our state-by-state guide or contact A Better Balance for more information on workplace leave and LGBT rights in your state.

Even if she can't care for me, can my same-sex partner take FMLA leave to care for our new baby?

Yes. Your partner can take FMLA leave to care for your newborn or seriously ill child even if she is not legally or biologically related to the child, and even if your marriage is not recognized in your state. The Department of Labor recently clarified that an LGBT parent who is raising a child is eligible to take FMLA leave to bond with or care for that child. So as long as your partner plays the role of a parent to the child, she can take FMLA leave to care for him or her.

If you and your partner or spouse work for the same employer, however, there may be limits on how many weeks of leave you can take altogether.

Getting Paid: Using Paid Time Off While on FMLA Leave

Can I use paid time off that I've earned on the job while on FMLA leave?

Yes, you can. This will enable you to earn some money while out on FMLA leave. There are limitations to using paid sick leave, however. Your use of sick leave must follow employer policy, as described in the next question.

Can my employer make me use my paid time off (including vacation) during my leave?

Yes, they can make you use saved-up, paid time off, such as vacation, but they do have to pay you for that time. However, your employer cannot force you to use paid sick leave if the employer's policy would forbid you from using those paid sick days. For example, if your employer does not allow you to take sick leave to care for children or a spouse, then they cannot force you to use your paid sick leave for your FMLA leave if you are using it to care for someone else. However, if you live in a state that requires employers to let you use your sick leave for "kin care," such as California, then the employer would have to follow that law.

Can I save any of my paid time off to use after my FMLA leave?

You might be able to if your employer does not require you to use your paid time off during FMLA leave. For example, you might want to take twelve weeks of unpaid leave and then two weeks of paid leave that you have saved. Your employer is allowed to say no to this plan and require you to be paid two weeks of the twelve weeks you are gone. Since you would like fourteen weeks off, hopefully you can negotiate with your employer for a satisfactory result.

What if I am entitled to disability benefits or state family leave benefits? Do these also run at the same time as my FMLA leave?

Your employer may designate disability leave as FMLA leave, but since disability leave is paid, you cannot substitute your own accrued paid time off for your disability leave. That means you can't decide that you'd rather use your paid sick days than your disability leave because the sick days pay more. However, if your employer agrees, and if your state law allows, you may use some paid leave to supplement your disability benefits. So if your temporary disability benefits add up to only about half of your regular salary, your employer can pay you while you are on disability leave to make up the difference. Just be careful about how you are paid because in some states, such as New York, for example, you may not receive paid sick leave at the same time as disability benefits. The law in New York considers sick time to be a duplication of benefits.

Taking It One Day (or One Hour) at a Time: Intermittent FMLA Leave

What is "intermittent leave?"

Intermittent leave means taking FMLA leave in separate blocks of time instead of taking all twelve weeks at once. For example, someone could take off one day per month in order to attend to medical appointments for a serious illness.

When may I take my leave intermittently?

Whenever it is medically necessary or you have an emergency. If the leave is being used for planned medical treatment, then you have to try to schedule the treatment so that it does not excessively disrupt your employer's operations. For example, a retail worker shouldn't schedule a surgery for Black Friday if it could just as easily be scheduled for the following week.

Can I use intermittent leave if I can't come to work because of severe morning sickness?

Yes, the Department of Labor's regulations specifically state that "a pregnant employee may take leave intermittently for prenatal examinations or for her own condition, such as for periods of severe morning sickness." You do not need employer permission to use your leave on an intermittent basis for these purposes.

Can my employer shift my job duties while I am on intermittent leave?

Yes. Your employer is allowed to temporarily transfer you to another position that you are qualified for but that is better suited for someone who needs intermittent leave or a reduced schedule. For example, if there are two administrative assistant positions, and one requires answering the phones, but the other involves completing paperwork with no set deadline, then the employer could temporarily shift the worker to the position without deadlines. The job must have the same pay and benefits. Note that special rules apply to teachers.

Can I take intermittent leave after my baby's birth in order to bond with her?

Only if your employer agrees. Your employer can refuse to let you take bonding leave intermittently; in other words, you would have to use it all in one large chunk. Of course, this is not the case if you or your newborn child has a serious health condition. You do *not* need your employer's permission to care for a child with a serious health condition on an intermittent basis.

Doing Your Homework: Your Responsibilities When Requesting Leave

When do I have to tell my employer that I plan to take leave?

If the leave is foreseeable (like an expected birth), then you must tell your employer at least thirty days before taking the FMLA leave. If it is not foreseeable, then you have to tell your employer as soon as possible. For example, if your due date is March 1, but you unexpectedly go into labor in late January, then you do not need to provide thirty days' notice, but you should tell your employer as soon as you can.

What do I have to do to request leave?

When you first ask for leave, you do not even have to mention the FMLA. You can simply speak with your employer about taking leave for an FMLA-qualifying reason. For example, you might say, "I need to go to a prenatal doctor appointment next month." This triggers your eligibility for FMLA leave even though you might not have even known that you were eligible for FMLA leave because it is your employer's responsibility to educate you about your rights.

However, once you are trying to get FMLA leave for the same FMLA-qualifying condition for a second time, then you have to specifically reference the same condition (in other words, your pregnancy) or your need for FMLA leave. So, you might say,

"I need to come in late today because I have pregnancy-related nausea," or you might say, "I need FMLA leave next month for another appointment." Remember, though, that it might be wise to try to use as little FMLA leave as possible until you deliver your baby, if other leave options are available.

How much time do they have to respond to my request for leave?
Your employer has five business days to respond, unless there are circumstances that justify a longer response time.

What if I miss the deadline?
If you should have told your employer thirty days before taking leave and missed that deadline, then your employer can delay your FMLA leave until thirty days after you gave notice. However, this is only the case if the employer fulfilled its notice requirements by telling employees about the FMLA, such as posting about the law in the office.

Do I need a doctor's note to take FMLA leave?
If you are taking leave because of your own serious health condition or the illness of a family member, then yes, your employer may request medical certification of the illness. Even if your employer does not request certification before you take leave, he or she can later request certification if he or she has reason to doubt the appropriateness of your taking FMLA leave. Sometimes a doctor's note will be sufficient for medical certification, but many employers have their own medical certification forms for a doctor to fill out. Medical certification is something your employer can request even after you have already brought in a doctor's note.

You do not need to bring in a doctor's note—or even have had a prenatal appointment—before taking intermittent FMLA leave for pregnancy-related sickness. However, your employer may request medical certification at some point after you begin taking that leave.

Dealing with Blowback: Retaliation and Discrimination

I returned from my FMLA leave only to find that my annual bonus is being prorated for the time I was out of the office. Is that legal?

Maybe. It depends on how your employer treats the bonuses of other employees who take leave for other reasons. For example, if your employer does not prorate the bonuses of your coworkers based on their vacation, sick, and personal time, you can't be penalized for using your saved-up vacation, sick, and personal time while out on FMLA leave. Similarly, if another employee takes non-FMLA leave that is unpaid (let's say, a leave of absence for a few months to promote a book he just wrote), and he still receives his full annual bonus, then you must get yours too. On the other hand, if your employer prorates the annual bonuses of all employees who take unpaid leave, whether or not it's covered by the FMLA, but does not do that for employees on paid leave, that's legal.

I filed a complaint with the Department of Labor after my employer denied my FMLA leave. Ever since then, my boss has been treating me terribly. He says I'm not loyal because I filed a complaint. I'm worried I will be fired. Can they do that?

No, your employer may not retaliate against you for filing a charge. Even if you are not fired, your boss might be violating the law because he is discriminating against you for filing a complaint. Employers are not allowed to interfere with your rights under the FMLA. Unfortunately, many employers will still try to retaliate, even though it is illegal. It might be helpful to contact a lawyer or call a legal hotline or community group. An advocate who has experience with these issues may be able to help keep a hostile employer off your back during the complaint process—for example, by writing a letter to the employer.

I returned from maternity leave and was treated worse than I ever had been before I took time off. After a few months of being under the microscope at work, I was fired. Is this illegal?

Maybe. The FMLA prohibits an employer from discriminating against you because you exercised your rights under the law. This includes firing or demoting you because you took FMLA leave. However, it can be hard to prove that the negative treatment you received was *because* of your maternity leave. For example, it may be that your boss realized while you were out that she or he could afford to run the business without you. Or maybe she or he hired someone while you were on leave to fill in for you, and this person did the job well for less money. If your employer has a valid business reason for firing you, the firing may be legal, even if it happened after you returned from protected leave. Also, the longer the time between your protected activity (i.e., taking FMLA leave) and the negative action by your employer (i.e., the firing in this case), the harder it can be to prove that one caused the other.

When I came back from maternity leave, I found that our entire department had been restructured and my job duties are very different now, although I still have the same title and pay. Is that illegal?

It depends. The test is whether or not your employer would have taken the same action if you hadn't been on leave. For example, if a company was having budget problems and had to do company-wide layoffs, then someone who is on FMLA leave can be laid off the same as they would have been if they had been working. Similarly, if the department restructuring and job duty changes would have happened even if you had been at work everyday, then it's probably not illegal. On the other hand, if it's clear that your job duties only changed because you were out on leave, then that could be a violation of the FMLA.

HOW THE OTHER HALF LIVES–
LEAVE OPTIONS BEYOND THE FMLA

What if you are among the 50 percent of private-sector workers not covered by the FMLA? Then what? As we mentioned at the start of this chapter, there are state laws that may guarantee time off or cash benefits to help you manage the arrival of a new family member. Here we explain each type of law and how they interact, but because each state's law is a bit different, you will want to check our state-by-state guide for more details. You also may have to call a local lawyer or legal hotline for more information, given that the overlap of these laws can get pretty tricky.

Getting the Time Off

If you are not covered by the FMLA, you are not necessarily out of luck. States also have the power to guarantee parental leave. In fact, when the FMLA became the law of the land in 1993, thirty-four states, Puerto Rico, and Washington, DC, already had state-mandated leave policies. Of all the states, however, only

Wisconsin and Maine guaranteed employees temporary leave for a "full range of family crises," as opposed to just pregnancy or disability leave. The FMLA was passed to set a minimum requirement for leave that applies to both men and women across the country, but states can, and many do, provide more protection than the federal law.

State Family Medical Leave Laws

Ten states and the District of Columbia have laws that mirror the FMLA or expand on its protections. All of these laws provide unpaid time off from work for one or more family and self-care situations. Some states, such as Maine and Oregon, cover employers that are smaller than those covered by the FMLA (i.e., employers with fewer than fifty employees). Others, such as Minnesota and Connecticut, include workers who have worked fewer than 1,250 hours in the twelve months before taking leave. Still others, such as New Jersey and Vermont, offer leave to care for family members who are not covered under the FMLA, such as domestic and civil-union partners. Check out our state-by-state guide for more details about your home state and to see whether you might be covered by one of these laws.

If you live in a state with its own family leave law, do your research on how it interacts with the FMLA. For example, in New Jersey, if you are entitled to leave under both the FMLA and the New Jersey Family Leave Law, you have to take both types of leave at the same time, which means you would get no more than twelve weeks total time off. This might be the case if you are a father bonding with your new baby and you are eligible for both FMLA and New Jersey Family Leave. However, since the New Jersey law doesn't provide leave to care for your own illness or injury, a pregnant woman could use FMLA leave for doctor-ordered bed rest at the end of her pregnancy and then still have twelve weeks left of New Jersey Family Leave to use to bond with her new baby. That could mean up to a total of twenty-four weeks of job-protected leave.

Pregnancy Disability Leave

Even states that don't have a family and medical leave law may still require a minimum amount of unpaid leave for pregnancy- and childbirth-related disability (i.e., when a woman is unable to work while pregnant or after giving birth). For example, if you live in Iowa and work for an employer who has four or more employees, you may be eligible for up to eight weeks of pregnancy disability leave. This is true even if your employer doesn't have any leave policy or if you are not eligible for sick time because you have not accrued enough yet. In Iowa, your employer *still* must grant you as many as eight weeks off if you are unable to work because of your pregnancy, because of childbirth, or because of another related medical condition. In order to take this leave, you must tell your boss as soon as you can about needing time off, and your boss may ask for a doctor's note.

Remember, pregnancy and childbirth disability leave is different from bonding leave; the former is available only for the birth mother. So in Iowa, Jennifer may be entitled to up to eight weeks of pregnancy disability leave if she is carrying a child, but her wife Evelyn is not. Evelyn would need to figure out whether she is eligible for FMLA leave to take time off when the baby arrives. (See the earlier FMLA discussion for more details.) Check out our state-by-state guide to see whether you might be able to take pregnancy disability leave in your state.

TIME-OUT FOR OUTRAGE!

Parenting a new child should not be a game of chance, let alone one with potentially devastating consequences. Yet this is the reality for millions of Americans who have no access to paid maternity or paternity leave.

Here are just a few stories we've heard from real families about the financial impact of living in a country with no guaranteed paid parental leave.

"The financial consequences of taking maternity leave left me with a hardship from which, even two years later, I have not recovered . . . During my pregnancy, I increased my savings as much as possible to cover my expenses during maternity leave. However, as I watched my savings dwindle, I had to cut back on expenses in order to stay afloat until I returned to work in the fall. Unable to reduce the expenses associated with caring for my newborn daughter, I cut my personal grocery bill down to the bare essentials, restricting my caloric intake so much that I was unable to breastfeed my daughter . . . By the end of my daughter's first year of life, I had destroyed my credit rating, obliterated my savings, and endured a level of stress, anxiety, depression, and sorrow I never imagined would have characterized my life after such a joyous event like giving birth."

"It is horrible that the United States is significantly behind the rest of the world with maternity leave. I am a single mom and had complications before and after pregnancy. I used my entire life savings and had to go into my 401(k) to survive."

"I am a teacher and love working with children; however, due to the current economic climate, my husband and I cannot have a child of our own yet because I can't afford to take the days off to care for a newborn. It is disheartening."

"I have a premature baby in a NICU in Buffalo. Both my partner and I have lost income, and for the time being our family is torn apart while I stay here with the baby and my partner is forced to choose work over parenting, lest we lose our home. Working families should not be punished with lost income for doing the responsible thing and caring for a sick child."

Paying for It

We hope you are lucky enough to qualify for FMLA leave or some other unpaid leave under state law, which means you can safely take time off without fear of losing your job. But how do you pay for your expenses if your employer doesn't pay you while you are out? Money is the other big piece of the puzzle, and unfortunately there aren't many state laws to help. In this section we highlight the states where you may be eligible for cash benefits while on pregnancy disability, childbirth disability, or bonding leave.

State Temporary or Short-Term Disability Insurance Laws

Temporary or short-term disability insurance (for simplicity's sake, we'll call it TDI) provides some cash benefit to workers who become injured or ill off the job and are unable to work as a result. The benefits replace some of the money you would be earning if you were able to work. Pregnancy-related disabilities that are severe enough to prevent you from working (such as preeclampsia that requires bed rest) may qualify you for temporary disability benefits. In addition, most insurers consider some period of time after childbirth as disabling. This means you could be entitled to benefits for a month or more to help you pay the bills after the baby arrives. Generally speaking, you should be able to collect TDI benefits while on unpaid leave, as a way of funding your absence from work. You may be able to draw benefits even while out on paid leave, but you need to check with your employer or state insurance fund to be sure that is allowed. For example, in New York State, you cannot receive TDI benefits while also receiving paid sick leave from your employer.

Five states (California, Hawaii, New York, New Jersey, and Rhode Island) and Puerto Rico have laws on the books that require employers to provide temporary disability insurance to their employees. This means that your employer has to buy insurance, either through the state plan or through a private insurer, which you may collect when you become eligible. The benefit rate can vary significantly, depending on where you live. For example, in New York, the maximum benefit as of 2014 is only $170 per week, whereas in California, it is $1,075 per week! Even if your state does not require temporary disability insurance, your employer may choose to offer this benefit to its employees. Make sure to check your employee handbook or ask your boss if your employer offers short-term disability benefits. If your employer does offer short-term disability insurance for other employees—for example, those who hurt their backs—they must offer it to you as a pregnant woman too.

It's important to remember that temporary disability insurance benefits are different from maternity leave. The disability laws do *not* guarantee you your job or a similar job back the way family and medical leave laws do. If you are not covered by the FMLA, you may not count on returning to your job. If you are covered by the FMLA and receive disability benefits while out on FMLA leave, your job is protected for only up to twelve weeks. If your disability lasts longer than that, you might still be entitled to disability benefits, but not to your job. Your employer could fire you at that point. It's true that your employer may not retaliate against you for taking FMLA leave (see the FMLA section above—Dealing with Blowback: Retaliation and Discrimination) and also may be prohibited from retaliating against you for claiming disability benefits under state law. In each case, however, you have to prove that your employer fired you *because* you tried to assert your rights by requesting leave or disability benefits, and it can be difficult to show that connection. There may be other laws that prohibit firing a worker in your situation (see chapter 4) that require proving discrimination. If you find yourself in the situation of losing your job after returning from disability or family leave, it's a good idea to consult an attorney about the strength of your case and your options.

State Family Leave Insurance Laws

If you are lucky enough to work in California, New Jersey, or Rhode Island you may be eligible to receive paid family-leave insurance benefits while you are bonding with your baby. Unlike temporary disability benefits, family leave insurance is available to men and women, to birth mothers and their partners. Both California and New Jersey provide up to six weeks of partial pay for workers to bond with a new baby. Like temporary disability benefits, these states' family leave insurance benefits do *not* come with job protection, but you may have access to that through your state's family leave or pregnancy leave laws. (See our state-by-state guide for more details.) Rhode Island provides up to four weeks of leave to bond with a new child or care for a seriously ill relative, and does offer job protection under the state Temporary Caregiver Insurance program.

Washington State also passed a paid family leave law in 2007, but the law has not yet been put into effect because of budget shortfalls.[17] The law would guarantee employees up to five weeks of benefits when they take time off work to care for a newborn or newly adopted child. If you live or work in Washington, keep your ears open for news about this benefit and when it might become a reality for your family.

Spotlight on the FAMILY Act

Nationwide, only 11 percent of private-sector workers have access to paid family leave and that number is even smaller–just 5 percent–for low-wage workers who are least likely to have the savings to weather weeks of lost pay.[18] Senator Kirsten Gillibrand (NY) and Representative Rosa DeLauro (CT) have introduced legislation to provide workers across the country with up to twelve weeks of partial income when they miss work to care for themselves, a seriously ill relative, or a new child. Not only would paid leave improve family health outcomes but it would also meaningfully contribute to economic productivity and growth.

"With benefits to both businesses and families, it is clear that even in an ongoing economic recovery, providing paid family and medical leave insurance is the right thing to do. In order for US companies to remain competitive, we must embrace smart policies like this one, which is a winner for the economy, business, and workers."

–Tom Nides, vice chairman, Morgan Stanley

"A large number of studies show that childcare, flexible work hours, and paid family leave all have a very high return on investment (ROI). Moreover, there is compelling evidence that points to the fact that companies can measurably improve their bottom line by transforming a company's corporate culture into one of a truly caring organization–which basically means, putting the interests of their employees first!"

–Cynthia D. DiBartolo, Esq., CEO Tigress Financial Partners LLC and chairperson, Greater New York Chamber of Commerce

---

To sum up, you may have additional maternity and paternity leave options available to you at the state law level, so it's important to do your homework! It's also important to realize that where you live and where you work can have an enormous impact on your well-being and that of your baby and family. Here's an example that may get you thinking about moving (or at least commuting) to New Jersey!

Keisha and Lily are neighbors and best friends living in Washington Heights in Manhattan, New York. They met in graduate school and are both social workers. Keisha works in Newark, New Jersey, for an after-school program that focuses on children with special needs. Lily works for a domestic violence shelter in Queens. Much to their surprise, the two friends get pregnant around the same time and have the exact same due date! Since neither woman's employer has an official maternity leave policy, the two women decide to spend a Saturday afternoon figuring out what the law guarantees them so that they will be armed with knowledge and can negotiate with their bosses in the following weeks.

Lily working in New York	**Keisha working in New Jersey**
Since Lily works in Queens, which is a borough of New York City, she must look at New York laws.	Even though Keisha is Lily's neighbor, her employer is in New Jersey, so she is covered by an entirely different set of laws.
Lily finds out that she is not covered by the FMLA since the shelter employs only thirty people.	Keisha also is not covered by the FMLA because the school where she is based has forty employees, and the next closest school in the network is in Camden, New Jersey, more than seventy-five miles away.
New York does not have a state family leave law, so Lily is not entitled to any job-protected time off to bond with her baby.[19]	Keisha is covered by the New Jersey Family Leave Act because her employer has over fifty employees, including its other locations in New Jersey and around the country. She is eligible for up to twelve weeks of leave to bond with her new baby.

Lily working in New York (*continued*)	**Keisha working in New Jersey** (*continued*)
Lily can receive temporary disability insurance payments (maximum of twenty-six weeks) when her pregnancy prevents her from working and for five to seven weeks after giving birth (depending on whether she has a vaginal birth or a C-section.) She can get up to **$170 per week**, depending on her salary.	Keisha also has access to New Jersey's temporary disability insurance (TDI) law. She can claim benefits while pregnant and while recovering from childbirth as long as she is unable to work (up to twenty-six weeks). She may receive up to **$572 per week**, depending on her salary.
New York doesn't have a family leave insurance program, so Lily won't be able to take advantage of it.	Keisha can use family leave insurance for up to six weeks to bond with her new baby. She gets part of her salary, but no more than **$572 per week**. She can claim these benefits as soon as her TDI benefits end, with no interruption in payment.

Lily is upset. "I thought New York was a liberal state! We have same-sex marriage, but pregnant women are worse off than New Jerseyians."

Keisha says, "I had no idea. I'd thought about moving to New Jersey for the lower rent, but I never thought my maternity leave would be so much better working there."

Lily responds, "Do you think they're hiring in Finland?"

CHECKLIST FOR MATERNITY AND PATERNITY LEAVE

Phew! And you thought the FMLA was complicated? Now that we've looked at a variety of state laws that might cover you, let's review the whole maternity/parental leave legal picture and how you plan to talk about this with your boss or human resources manager. Your employer may know a lot about these laws we've discussed, or they may know very little. In order to be your own best advocate, you need to know the legal landscape before you start the conversation.

1. ***Figure out whether you are covered by the FMLA.*** If you are eligible for FMLA leave, start thinking about whether you can afford to take twelve weeks unpaid. If not, see how many paid days off you have accrued and save them for your leave. Also, think about whether you might want to take any leave intermittently after your baby is born. If so, come up with a plan about how to handle your work while you transition back into full-time work.
2. ***Do your state research.*** Start with our state-by-state guide to see whether you might be entitled to any additional time off or wage replacement through state law. Are you a state employee? If so, state law may guarantee you some additional parental leave benefits. Consult your local state agencies for more information as to how the laws apply to your situation. You also may want to bring printed information (such as your state's page[s] from our state-by-state guide) to your meeting with your boss, given that she or he may not know much about these local laws.
3. ***Review your employee handbook.*** Employers all have different policies, so it's best to check what your employer has

put in writing. Some things to look out for: Does your company offer any paid time off for maternity? What is the pay rate during maternity leave? How much maternity leave time is available to you? What about paternity leave? What does your health insurance cover? Sometimes policies are not written down, so it can help to talk with other employees who have been pregnant or have had children while working for your employer.

4. ***Check your union contract.*** If you are a union member, check your union contract and talk with your union representative because you may be entitled to more leave or other protections under the contract. Some unions use collective bargaining to gain better work–life policies for their members. For examples, check out our list of resources.
5. ***Do some comparative research.*** If there is no policy on the books and no guidance from others' past experience, you may find yourself blazing the trail. Before you begin your negotiation with your employer, try to find out what other employers like yours provide and see whether you can find industry- and size-specific information. For helpful data sources, check out our resources on page 183.
6. ***Plan ahead.*** Think about how you can put yourself in the best position for pregnancy and beyond. You may have to use paid time off that you've earned on the job for your maternity leave, so it's best to start saving that time in advance as much as you can. Try to find a doctor who has extended office hours, so that you don't have to miss work for your prenatal appointments and can save your precious time off for post-baby leave. Make sure your partner does his or her research too because your partner's work may offer different (and maybe even more generous) benefits.

We know we are giving you a lot to think about while you are dealing with the other challenges and thrills of pregnancy. But doing this work up front and as early as you can means more time to focus on your new family after the baby arrives. Before you know it, you'll be returning to work! That's what our next chapter is all about.

TOP FIVE THINGS TO REMEMBER

- The United States has no federal law guaranteeing paid maternity leave.
- The Family and Medical Leave Act guarantees unpaid time off to care for yourself, a new baby, or a seriously ill family member and protects your job while you are gone. But not all workers are covered by the FMLA.
- Going out on temporary disability does not necessarily mean that your job will be open for you when you are ready to work again.
- Fathers and same-sex partners can use FMLA leave to bond with and care for a new child, but same-sex partners may not be able to use the FMLA to care for their pregnant partners.
- You may use FMLA leave on a sporadic basis to deal with morning sickness and other pregnancy-related health reasons.

3 BACK INTO THE GROOVE
Returning to Work as a Parent

• POP QUIZ •

True or False?

1. **Employers can make all nursing employees pump their breast milk in the bathroom.**
   False. If the employee is covered by the Federal Labor Standards Act (don't worry; we'll go over this), then she is entitled to pump in a private space other than the bathroom.

2. **Everyone gets three paid sick days per year that they can use to care for their kids.**
   False. There are actually no federal laws that make employers give you paid sick days, and there are only limited local laws that might provide paid sick time.

3. **Under US law, workers have the right to request a flexible work arrangement without penalty.**
   False. Unlike in the United Kingdom and other countries, there are no legal protections guaranteeing you this right. Instead, your employer calls the shots.

So you took a little time away from work and now are ready to get back to the grind (or maybe you aren't ready, but you need some money—diapers don't grow on dogwoods, after all). Not getting spit-up on your suit and eliminating the semipermanent bags under your eyes seem like enough of a challenge, so how can you figure out your rights in the workplace during such a busy time?

In this chapter we talk about how you might have a right to pump breast milk at work, a right to a reduced or flexible schedule (pretty rare), a right to use sick time to care for your child, or a right to keep your job after returning from maternity leave. Of course, these are all "maybes" or even "probably nots," but if you can't jump right back into eighty-hour workweeks, then read on!

NURSING ON THE JOB

If you're a nursing mother, chances are you'd like to continue breastfeeding when you return to work. Many of you value the health benefits that breastfeeding provides to you and your baby and will have just gotten into a groove.[20]

Unfortunately, many working mothers have to stop breastfeeding because it's not possible to pump milk at work.

> **After years of hard work and training, Melissa was close to graduating from a prestigious medical school. She had a new baby and only six and a half weeks of leave to recover before she had to return to her residency program. Her newborn needed to feed every four hours, so Melissa asked for twenty minutes of break time every few hours so that she could pump milk for her baby. Her clinic director made her pump in an unlocked room,**

where someone could walk in on her at any moment, and then in a toilet stall. He further punished her by deducting her break time from her vacation leave and making her work extra hours to make up for time her "time off." He told Melissa, "If a patient with a colostomy bag can train his bowels to shit at regular hours, then you can train your boobs to pump after-hours."

Yes, this is a *true* story from the medical profession. Hard to believe, huh? However, most of the horror stories we hear are from low-wage women in hourly work. Inflexible workplaces, unsanitary conditions, and unsupportive managers have all factored into a woman's decision to stop breastfeeding after returning to work.

The good news is that the government thinks it's a good idea to breastfeed your baby and wants to support you. A new federal law says you have the right to breastfeed your baby at work, and you must get break time and a protected space to do it.

Nursing Moms' Rights in a Nutshell

WHAT?

The Affordable Care Act (President Obama's health care law) requires employers to provide "reasonable break time for an employee to express breast milk for her nursing child for one year after the child's birth each time such employee has need to express the milk." Employers are also required to provide "a place, other than a bathroom, that is shielded from view and free from intrusion from coworkers and the public, which may be used by an employee to express breast milk."

WHO?

The law applies to employers and employees covered under the Fair Labor Standards Act (FLSA), the law that sets minimum wage and overtime requirements. FLSA-exempt employees (e.g., administrative and professional workers) are *not* covered by this law but may be protected by state breast-feeding laws, as indicated in our state-by-state guide. Exempt employees who work for federal government agencies *are* covered by the law. Employers who have fewer than fifty employees *and* who would have significant difficulty complying with the law because of their size, their financial resources, or the nature or structure of their business *may* be excluded. To see whether you qualify as a nonexempt worker, visit http://www.dol/gov/compliance/guidance/minwage.htm.

WHEN?

Assuming your employer is covered, they must provide *reasonable unpaid break time* for you to express breast milk, each time you need to pump, for up to one year after you give birth. You should get a break about as often as you would feed your baby if you were with him or her. The length of your breaks will depend on how long it takes to get to your pumping space, the speed of your pump, and other factors. Finally, if your employer provides paid breaks, you must be allowed to use that paid time to pump milk.

WHERE?

In addition, your employer must give you a clean, private space, *other than a bathroom*, where you can pump milk with no interruption. Your employer may create a temporary or converted space for you to use while expressing milk, as long as it is protected from coworkers and the public and is available to you whenever you need it. The space must be functional as a space to pump breast milk. Finally, breaks for expressing breast milk do not qualify as family or medical leave and should not be counted against your entitlement to such leave. Also, your employer can't fire you for taking breaks you are entitled to under the law.

ANYTHING ELSE?

Not only does the ACA protect the right to breastfeed in the workplace, it also requires many health care plans to provide breastfeeding help to new moms at no cost. Women enrolled in any health plan through a state or federal exchange, as well as many other health plans, can get comprehensive lactation support and counseling by a trained provider during and/or after pregnancy without a co-payment or deductible. Your health insurance plan must also provide you with breastfeeding equipment, including a breast pump, at no cost. Health plans may offer either a rental pump, or a new one for you to keep. Some "grandfathered" health plans that were created on or before March 23, 2010, are exempt from these provisions of the Affordable Care Act, so call your insurance company to ask whether these rules apply to your plan.

WHAT THE LAW DOES NOT COVER:

Although we are making progress in support of nursing mothers, we are not where we need to be. These new rules in the Affordable Care Act cover only "nonexempt" workers and not those who have salaried positions, such as a staff attorney or an accountant. As a result, approximately half of new mothers are unprotected. (Some states do provide greater protection than federal law, so check our state-by-state guide.)

What should I do if I think my rights have been violated?

Call the US Department of Labor's Wage and Hour Division, toll-free, at 1-866-487-9273. They can help you file a complaint and investigate your claim.

If you think you've been discriminated against as a nursing mother, contact the Equal Employment Opportunity Commission at 1-800-669-4000 or visit the commission's website, http://www.eeoc.gov/employees.

For more general information about your rights under the new breast-feeding law, please visit http://www.dol/gov/whd/nursingmothers.

When should I tell my employer I want to keep breast-feeding at work?

There are no requirements. Legally, you can return to work and tell your employer then that you need a time and space to express breast milk, and they must try to accommodate you, if you are covered. However, if you intend to breast-feed and return to work, you're best off initiating a conversation with your supervisor during your pregnancy. Many employers are happy to support you if they know what you need and why it's important to you. Don't assume that because your employer does not have a formal lactation policy or designated pumping room, you're out of luck. Remember, providing the time and space to pump breast milk is the law for many workers.

What should I say?

The conversation should make the following points:[21]

1. Breast-feeding is the healthiest choice for you and your baby, resulting in fewer illnesses and infections, and may reduce your risk of breast cancer.
2. Your breast-feeding will benefit the company.
   — Employees who breast-feed are less likely to miss work to take care of a sick baby because the baby is healthier.

- — Health care costs are lower since both baby and mother are healthier.
- — Employees who receive support for breast-feeding are happier and more productive.[22]

Explain that you are committed to keeping the milk-expression area clean when you are through, to storing milk properly, and to not taking longer than necessary for milk-expression breaks.

Be prepared! Consider possible concerns that your supervisor might have. If your supervisor says they do not have space for pumping, look around and find a space you are willing to use. Even a small space can work! And if your employer says they can't make an exception for one employee, remind him or her that breast-feeding benefits the company and is the law. Also, remind your supervisor of other company-approved breaks, such as those for smoking or exercise, if offered.

Sample Letter to Your Supervisor[23]

TO: [Supervisor's name]
FROM: [Your name]
RE: Lactation support in the workplace

First, I want to thank you for your support during my [number] years with [company]. This is an exciting time for my family as we prepare for the birth of our child. I am eager to work with you to assure my productive return to work as soon as practicable after the birth of my baby.

Based on advice from my doctor and other health professionals, I have made the decision to breast-feed my baby. Just as I want to continue to give my best to the company, I also want to give the best I can to my baby. My doctor tells me that breast-feeding is important in preventing illness and diseases for my baby and for me. Many employers across America now help make breast-feeding possible for working mothers. I hope we can find a mutually beneficial way to make breastfeeding possible when I am back at work.

If the company has an established lactation policy, I would like to know what it is so I can begin planning. If you want to understand better what is involved, you may want to start by looking at www.worksitesforwellness.org/for-employers.htm.

Thank you. Knowing that the company will help make it possible for me to continue breast-feeding will make me feel much better about leaving my baby at home to come back to work. I look forward to discussing this with you.

[your signature]

What if I am not covered by federal law?

Because the Affordable Care Act's breast-feeding provisions only apply to certain classes of workers, many mothers still find themselves without any legal right to express breast milk at work. That's what happened to this public school teacher who called us from Wisconsin:

> **Rebecca's baby boy was born three-and-a-half months premature. When Rebecca returned from maternity leave, she wanted to continue pumping breast milk to provide her son with sufficient nutrition and critical antibodies to protect his vulnerable immune system as flu**

season approached. But her schedule required her to work from 7:30 a.m. until noon without a break. In order to maintain milk supply for her son, she needed to pump more often, so she asked her employer for a mid-morning break to express milk. The school said no, and told her to wait until her lunch break to pump. But waiting such an extended time between feedings lead to severe discomfort and caused her milk supply to drop. Rebecca was able to get other teachers to cover her class recess for a while, so she could sneak in a pumping session, but her colleagues were less willing to stand out in the cold to do her a favor as winter set in. And despite her best efforts to find other workable solutions, her employer was unwilling to budge.

Almost half the states have their own laws protecting a woman's right to express breast milk at work. Check our state-by-state guide to see if your state is among those with additional protections. If not, don't give up! You may be able to convince your employer to help you continue pumping at work by using some of our resources on page 183.

EASING BACK IN—WHAT IF YOU NEED MORE TIME?

If there's one thing we've learned from hearing stories in our clinic, it's that every woman truly is different. Some have had difficult pregnancies and traumatic childbirths. For them the idea of returning to work a mere twelve weeks after bearing a child is unthinkable. On the other hand getting back to the grind three days after giving birth might be no problem! Whatever your situ-

TIME-OUT FOR OUTRAGE!

Did you know that 163 other countries around the world guarantee workers some number of paid sick days and that 155 countries provide a week or more paid sick time per year? This is yet another area where the United States stands alone compared to other developed and many developing countries. Most workers in the United States have *no legal guarantee of paid sick time* to deal with their own illness or to care for a child or other family member. Even if *you* get sick time through your employer, chances are high that the person next to you on the subway or the waiter serving your salad or the day care worker taking care of your child does not. This is a serious public health problem!

Also, because the United States does not guarantee paid parental leave, plenty of expecting parents come to work sick in order to save their sick time for maternity or paternity leave. Here's one all-too-common story from New York:

> "A pregnant coworker of my partner keeps coming to work right now, even though she has a bad cold. She is doing so to save up her sick days because her employer, a nonprofit, only offers one week of maternity leave. This is just wrong. It's bad for her, for babies in NY State, and for my partner who has to deal with working with a sick coworker."

ation, you might be wondering about any right you have to time off now that your screaming bundle of joy has arrived.

Postpartum Depression and Other Disabilities

The Centers for Disease Control and Prevention estimates that between 10 and 15 percent of mothers report postpartum depression symptoms.[24] If you suffer from postpartum depression, you might be protected by the Americans with Disabilities Act (see chapter 1—Workplace Accommodations for Complicated or Difficult Pregnancies—for more information). This federal law not only protects workers from being discriminated against because of their disabilities; it also lets you ask your boss for the help you need to get the job done. Part-time work or some time off could be a solution to help you get better while keeping you on the job. If your boss doesn't want to accommodate your depression, or any other physical or mental disabilities you might have, consider discussing your options with a lawyer.

Intermittent Leave/Flexible Return to Work

You might be thinking about part-time work or other flexible options. We discuss flexible work schedules in greater detail later in this chapter, but first we want you to know that the FMLA may be able to help.

If you qualify to take time off under the Family and Medical Leave Act (see chapter 2—Are You In or Out? Who Is Covered under the FMLA?—for more details), then you might be able to use the law to help you ease back into the workforce. As we discussed in chapter 2, the FMLA (which applies to only about half of American workers, so double-check your eligibility status) allows you to take twelve weeks in a twelve-month period, either all at once or in smaller chunks.

Someone who had a healthy pregnancy could have all her FMLA time remaining after giving birth. She would then have twelve weeks for what the law calls "bonding" with her baby. Fathers, non–birth mothers, and adoptive parents get "bonding" time as well. These twelve weeks can be used all at once, but for many parents, going three months without a paycheck is not an affordable option. A better option might be using a little bit of leave at a time, such as working part-time for twenty-four weeks or working out another arrangement. FMLA leave may be taken in this way, but *only if the employer agrees to it*. (However, you do not need your employer's agreement if you have a "serious health condition" connected to the birth of the child or if your newborn has a serious health condition. Take a look at chapter 2—Taking It One Day (or One Hour) at a Time: Intermittent FMLA Leave—for more information on taking a little leave at a time, which is called "intermittent leave.")

Here's a hypothetical example of how intermittent FMLA leave could work.

> **Maria gave birth a month ago but is going crazy worrying about her big account back at the office. She asks her boss if she can come back to work part-time and use the remaining eight weeks of her FMLA leave time to take off the afternoons so that she can be with her son. For sixteen weeks she would work half the time. Her boss agrees.**

This is a legal way to use FMLA time after the baby is born. Maria's boss still has to comply with other FMLA requirements. For example, he can't fire her for taking the FMLA time off.

Sick Time to Care for a Sick Child

What if you are back at work, but your baby gets an ear infection or needs to go in for her three-month checkup? Pre-baby, you might have been the type of employee who never took a sick day, either because you were extremely healthy or because you always powered through the sniffles. But it's different when your little one comes down with a nasty bug. Not only will day cares and schools reject sick children and make them stay home, but you might need to take them in to the doctor.

The first step is to review your employer's policies about sick time or personal time off. Does your employer let you take sick

PAID SICK LEAVE

What if you don't get sick days at all, for yourself or to care for others? Only about 58 percent of private-sector workers have sick days, and in some areas of the country, that number is even lower. There's a small chance your employer is breaking the law by not providing sick days because there are a few cities (and one state, Connecticut) that require some employers to provide paid sick leave to their employees. Again, check your state in the guide at the end of this book. If you think you deserve paid sick leave because of where you live and who your employer is, contact a lawyer. Keeping yourself healthy is important too!

days when a child is ill? What about personal days? If you have a partner, have your partner check his or her policies at work as well. You might be surprised to learn that you cannot use sick time to care for a sick child. If so, you are in the majority: about 70 percent of workers who have sick time cannot use it to care for their children when they are ill.

If this is the case, check to see whether your state has what is called a "kincare law" (see our state-by-state guide). These laws enable workers to use sick leave or other paid leave to care for sick family members, including children.

If all these options fall short, try to negotiate with your boss and talk to coworkers. Is there a sick leave pool available in your office? Can you trade shifts? Will your boss let you work late sometime to make up for any hours missed? Hopefully someone will be able to help you out.

You might be thinking that some of the laws we have talked about should help a parent with a sick kid (such as the Americans with Disabilities Act or the Family and Medical Leave Act). You are right—there's a chance, but probably not for a run-of-the-mill cold or routine checkup for a healthy child. Remember that the ADA applies only to disabilities, although that includes some temporary disabilities, and the FMLA applies only to "serious medical conditions." However, state law might entitle you to additional leave for routine medical appointments. For example, the Massachusetts Small Necessities Leave Act entitles qualifying employees to twenty-four hours of unpaid leave per year, which they can use to accompany a child to routine medical or dental appointments. Check your state's laws to be sure.

Spotlight on New York City Earned Sick Time Act

If you are one of the 3.4 million private-sector workers in New York City, you are in luck! On April 1, 2014, the New York City Earned Sick Time Act went into effect. This landmark law ensures that workers in New York City can take time off for personal or family health needs without losing their jobs, and provides *paid* sick time to many of these workers. Here's an overview of what the law provides:

- All private-sector workers, even those in the smallest businesses, cannot be punished or fired for taking up to 40 hours of unpaid sick time per year.
- Private-sector workers in businesses with 5 or more employees will earn one hour of paid sick time for every 30 hours worked, and they will be able to earn up to 40 hours of paid sick time per year. The law covers full-time, part-time, and most temporary workers.
- Domestic workers in New York City will be entitled to two paid sick days in addition to the "days of rest" they receive under state law.
- Paid or unpaid sick time can be used to care for a worker's own health needs or to care for the health needs of a worker's spouse, domestic partner, child, parent, grandparent, grandchild, siblings, or the child or parent of a worker's spouse or domestic partner.
- Any type of paid leave a worker already gets, such as paid vacation or personal days, will count for purposes of complying with the law as long as it can be used under the same conditions and for the same purposes as the Earned Sick Time Act.

CHILD CARE: WHAT ARE YOUR OPTIONS?

Although this issue is not the focus here, we couldn't write a whole book about becoming a working parent without mentioning child care. The challenge of investigating child care programs, nannies, co-ops, and other arrangements can be enough to make any new parent cower in fear. We could probably draft dozens of pages just on this topic! Instead, we simply want to flag a few key issues for you so that you can do your own research about options in your area.

Here in America, almost all laws and policies about child care apply at the state and local levels. Child care laws usually come in the form of tax credits or subsidies of some sort (in addition to regulations on child care centers and family child care homes themselves). And child care sure is expensive! Costs can range from $4,000 to over $15,000 a year.[25] High-quality care in urban areas can be much more expensive than that. In fact, at every income level, child care costs are among the top three expenses for families, right up there with housing, food, and transportation.[26] Our government does not defray much of the cost and most of the aid is directed toward low-income families. Some parents also receive financial assistance from other sources, such as their employers or family members.[27]

Contrast this picture to the one in France, where even before entering school, children have access to early childhood care.[28] Some children between two and a half months and three years attend government-subsidized child care programs (crèches) where fees are based on household income and region.[29] Daycare workers in France are also well-trained and paid better than workers in the United States.[30] Parents can also opt to hire a caregiver in-house and receive tax breaks, often amounting to about one-third the total cost of care.[31] For all children between three and six years old, prekindergarten programs (the *ecole maternelle*) are available. Over 95 percent of eligible three- to six-year-olds attend these schools because they are essentially free and high quality.[32] No wonder moms in France make it look so easy!

Child Care Assistance

The US government provides child care assistance for some low-income families. The federal Child Care and Development Block Grant gives $5.2 billion to states for child care subsidies so that low-income parents can go to work or school.[33] The funds are also used for improving the quality of child care.[34] Although the federal government provides the bulk of the funding, states can pretty much use the money as they see fit. States can also use funds from the Temporary Assistance for Needy Families (TANF) program, which is what public assistance (formerly welfare) is called, to help pay for child care subsidies for families in need.[35] States can have different policies about how much money you can make and still qualify for subsidies, other eligibility requirements, waiting lists, copayments required of parents, and reimbursement rates for child care providers.[36] You will have to look at your state government's website to understand the requirements of your particular state. Unfortunately, because of a lack of funding, only one in six children who are eligible for assistance under federal law is currently receiving it.[37] This means that even if you are low-income, you might not be able to count on assistance from the government in the form of child-care subsidies.

Tax Credits

You might be able to claim the Child and Dependent Care Credit on your federal tax income returns in order to help defray the high cost of child care.[38] If you spend money on care for a child under thirteen years old so that you can work, then you could qualify for a tax credit.[39] This can be up to $3,000 spent in one year for one child or up to $6,000 for two or more children in child care.[40] Many states also provide their own tax credits or deductions for child care expenses. In a number of states, the credit is refundable.[41] Talk to an accountant to try to find out whether your family qualifies for a tax credit or deduction and for how much.

Head Start

You have probably heard of Head Start. Head Start helps primarily low-income children from birth to five years old.[42] Over one million children are a part of Head Start each year.[43] Early Head Start is for children from birth to three years old, and Head Start is for children ages three to five.[44] Head Start is not just preschool; it also includes healthy meals, access to health and dental care, and support for parents.[45] In terms of what Head Start looks like, most children attend half days at a center, although sometimes full-day programs or home-based programs are available.[46] Unfortunately, Head Start helps only about two-fifths of eligible three- and four-year-olds and less than 3 percent of eligible children up to three years old.[47]

State-Funded Prekindergarten

Preschool can be public or private, just like other schools. Thirty-two percent of four-year-olds and 8 percent of three-year-olds used state-funded prekindergarten programs in 2011.[48] Thirty-nine states have programs, although thirty-one have an income requirement.[49] Recent budget cuts are undermining programs' ability to bring quality care and keep up with rising demand from families whose incomes have fallen in the latest recession.[50] Circumstances have varied state by state, and it might not all be bad news, so be sure to check out the local prekindergarten programs available to you.

Quality Rating and Improvement Systems

As of January 2012, twenty-six states have quality rating and improvement systems (QRIS).[51] These are used to rate the quality of child care centers and sometimes family child care homes, to provide incentives for programs to improve quality, and to offer parents information about the quality of programs.[52] States are different in how they implement their systems, but one goal is to provide information to parents so that they can find high-quality child care. Parents do not always receive additional assistance to purchase the higher quality care.

The takeaway from this section is that most child care assistance is for low-income families, and even those families who are eligible often can't take advantage of the benefits because of a shortage of funding. For a middle-class family investigating quality child care options and trying to make ends meet, it can be frustrating to find out there aren't many programs to suit their needs.

Many parents turn to their families and communities for help, since governmental policies usually come up short. Policymakers need to work to make sure that existing programs are given appropriate funding and to expand current programs to ensure that more children have access to high-quality care. After all, parents should not have to choose between having a job and their child's safety and well-being.

The New York State Domestic Workers Bill of Rights

If you live in New York and employ a domestic worker (a nanny, housecleaner, etc.) or are yourself a domestic worker, then you should know about the Domestic Workers Bill of Rights (DWBOR). Even if you don't live in New York, it is still helpful to understand some bare minimum guidelines for how employers should treat domestic workers. After all, everyone wants those working in the home to be happy and healthy!

Under this statewide law, domestic workers are entitled to the following:

- At least one full day of rest each week (i.e., twenty-four hours)
- At least three paid days off each year, after one year of work for you
- Guaranteed wage of at least $7.25 per hour (New York State minimum wage)
- Overtime pay of one and one-half the regular hourly rate after forty hours of work per week or after forty-four hours for live-in employees. Employees also get time and a half if they work on their day of rest

(Note: this is not an exhaustive list. To learn more, visit www.abetterbalance.org. Domestic workers can also get more information about their rights from the National Domestic Workers Alliance at www.domesticworkers.org.)

FINDING YOUR BALANCE: GETTING THE WORK SCHEDULE YOU WANT

Flexible Work Arrangements

As your parental leave winds down (if you're fortunate enough to have one!) and you begin planning your return to work, you may have mixed emotions. You may be dreaming of more time with your baby and dreading your long workweek and difficult commute. Before you call it quits in your sleep-deprived state, realize that it doesn't necessarily have to be all or nothing. With careful thought and planning, you may be able to create a new work arrangement that allows you more flexibility in how, when, and where work gets done.

Flexible work arrangements include:

- — adjustable work schedules, which include flexibility in the scheduling of hours worked, such as starting and stopping early or arrangements regarding shift and break schedules
- — predictable schedules, in which work schedules are provided with as much notice as possible and changes to work schedules are minimized once they are assigned
- — reduced hours, such as part-time work, job sharing, phased retirement, and part-year work
- — alternative locations, which provide flexibility in the place of work, such as working at home or at a satellite location[53]

Workplace flexibility is a proven "win-win" for employers and employees. Employers who provide flexibility to their employees, with regard to where and how their work gets done, gain a tremendous financial benefit and competitive advantage in today's economy. Overwhelming data has shown that workplace flexibility is a crucial tool in recruiting and retaining employees, reducing turnover, and enhancing productivity.[54] In fact, in March 2010, President Obama's Council of Economic Advisers issued a report exploring these benefits in depth.[55] Workplace flexibility also makes for happier, healthier workers—in fact, work–life balance is the second-best predictor, after economic security, of a worker's quality of health, frequency of sleep problems, and level of stress![56] And nearly a third of US workers consider work–life balance and flexibility to be the most important factor in considering job offers.

The Business Case for Flexible Work Practices[57]

Workplace flexibility is good not only for the health of employees but also for a business's bottom line. Here are some facts to get you started in convincing your employer to try out flexible policies:

Workplace flexibility is a powerful tool for recruiting and keeping the best employees.

- Almost three-quarters of workers said that the benefit of workplace flexibility would help them choose between job options.
- The vast majority of workers want flexible work options; in fact, 85 percent of younger workers want more flexibility at work.

- Many human resources managers name family-friendly workplace policies as the single most important factor in attracting and retaining employees.

Flexible work makes for happier, healthier workers.

- Employees in flexible workplaces have significantly better health than other employees.
- Stress is the leading cause of unscheduled absences and a factor in high turnover, but flexible work practices reduce stress.
- Caregiving responsibilities that interrupt work are estimated to cost employers billions of dollars each year.

Workplace flexibility increases productivity.

- Workers with flexibility have higher job satisfaction and are likely to feel like they have a stake in the organization.
- Senior-level corporate executives say that flexible work options help them meet their business goals.
- Research shows that flexibility increases productivity and shareholder returns.

However, there's an unfortunate reality—besides the breastfeeding and Family and Medical Leave Act and the Americans with Disabilities Act protections we just described, US law does little to guarantee you flexible work. In the United States, workplace flexibility is not an entitlement. Although some employers recognize the bottom-line benefits of flexible work, others remain stubbornly resistant. Far too many companies have good policies on paper but do little, if anything, to encourage employees to work flexibly. According to the Families and Work Institute, these companies cling to outdated assumptions, including the ideas that "presence equals productivity" and "if you give employees an inch, they'll take a mile."[58]

By contrast, the United Kingdom and many other countries actively encourage businesses and individuals to pursue family-friendly policies. For example, the United Kingdom's Flexible Working Act grants parents and other family caregivers the statutory *right to request* flexible working arrangements from their employers if they have been employed continuously for twenty-six weeks.[59] Under the law, an employer must seriously consider an employee's application for flexible work and can deny the request only if there are good business reasons for doing so. The government's official website is clear: Brits have the right to *apply* for flexible working, not the right to *have* it. However, by laying out a process for employees and employers to negotiate a mutually beneficial arrangement, the law has played an important role in helping to expand access to flexible work in the United Kingdom.[60] Score another one for the United Kingdom!

Flexible Work in the United States

In 2013, San Francisco and Vermont enacted laws like the one in the United Kingdom, granting certain workers the right to request flexible work arrangements without penalty. These are the first laws of their kind in the United States. San Francisco's law is limited to workers who request a flexible work arrangement to attend to their caregiving obligations for young children, aging parents or seriously ill relatives, whereas Vermont's law applies broadly to all workers. Both laws go into effect in 2014, and will allow employees to request alternative scheduling without fear of retaliation. Check out the state-by-state for more details.

Still, even though most employers are not required by law

to consider flexible work arrangements, many companies in the United States voluntarily recognize the business benefits of workplace flexibility and are willing to consider such arrangements. The ball is in your court to ask for one. This is where careful thought and planning come into play—without a solid and realistic proposal, your manager may reject your request on the spot. Are you worried because your employer is notoriously rigid? Have you not been around that long, or do you work in a low-wage or hourly job where flexible work arrangements are even harder to come by? Don't be discouraged. According to work–life expert Cali Yost in her excellent book *Work + Life: Finding the Fit That's Right for You*, successful flexibility isn't company-initiated and managed; it's employee-initiated and managed.[61] "Employees," she writes, "*must* be encouraged to create, negotiate and manage a work–life fit compatible with the tasks and responsibilities of their job and their work style."[62] In other words, the perfect flex job isn't going to fall in your lap—you need patience, vision, and a well-thought-out proposal to make it happen.

Tips for Proposing a Flexible Work Arrangement

Although there aren't any real legal requirements for requesting a flexible work schedule, there are some best practices you should know about. Ellen Galinsky, president and cofounder of the Families and Work Institute (FWI), is a pioneer in this field and has done the homework for you. In fact, we liked her advice so much we have reproduced it below verbatim. She and her colleagues recommend the following steps for finding a flexible work arrangement that helps you meet your work and family commitments: assess your situation, work on creating solutions, and make the

UNION MEMBERS

As a union member, you may have the right to flexible work through your collective bargaining agreement. Check with your union representative or request a copy of your union contract to see whether there are any provisions that might help you meet your work and family obligations. You might be entitled to make a gradual return from parental leave, for example, or to use sick time to care for family members. Or your union might negotiate for better policies, so tell them this is important to you.[63] Even for workers whose union contracts do not include such family-friendly protections, there is still good news: a study of union arbitrations involving work-family conflicts showed that arbitrators often do not rigidly enforce workplace rules when workers face discipline or discharge because of family care needs, so long as they have adequate child (or other) care and backup care in place.[64]

case for your proposal.[65] (We also highly recommend a new publication from When Work Works, a project of the FWI and Society for Human Resources Management [SHRM], which offers excellent tips and tools for making "workflex" a reality in your career.[66])

Assessing Your Situation

First, determine your needs for flexibility. Do you need or want traditional flextime, in which you select arrival and departure times and then stick with them? Or daily flextime, varying your arrival and departure times daily? Do you want to work at home occasionally or on a regular basis? Do you want to reduce your hours over the course of a week, or during certain times of the year? There are many types of workplace flexibility—for more information, go to www.whenworkworks.org.

Find out what kinds of flexibility your organization offers by talking to the people responsible for personnel policies, reading the employee handbook, and/or talking with other employees. Just because your company may not offer the kind of flexibility you need and want, doesn't mean you can't be the first person to pioneer it.

As you are considering the possibilities, think about your working style. If you are thinking of flextime, then make sure you can reliably stick to the schedule you select. If you are thinking of working from home, you should be a self-starter—able to take initiative, work independently, deal effectively with the distractions of home life, meet deadlines, and produce well.

If you are planning to work from home, make sure your home has a good space for working—where you can keep and store work materials and equipment. Consider whether you will need equipment, technology support, or other resources from the company to make your arrangement work.

You need to be realistic and think about the potential impact on you and your career. Could this arrangement affect your ability to advance in your career or be selected for specific work assignments? How will the flexible arrangement impact your income? How will it impact your eligibility in the short term for benefits such as health care coverage and in the long term for your retirement pension?

Creating Solutions

Consider how the flexible work arrangement you want will affect your job responsibilities, your company, customers, supervisors, and coworkers.

Talk with employees who have used flexible arrangements. Find out what's worked and what hasn't and how and when they involved their coworkers and supervisor. What advice would they give you? Use this information in shaping your own plan.

Create several options for handling your job responsibilities that will work well for you AND for your company, customers, supervisors, and coworkers. Plan for everyday and emergency situations. For example, if you want a flextime schedule where you come to work early and leave early, figure out how problems that arise after your departure will be handled. Make sure that these are realistic solutions that others can handle. Your supervisor is much more likely to be open to your proposal if he or she sees that you've given thought to your work, as well as your personal needs, and looked for win-win solutions.

Most important to any arrangement is a communications plan, i.e., the need to determine when, where, and how you will be available to your supervisor, coworkers, and clients. If you work part-time, job share, or are on a compressed workweek, you also need to decide on your accessibility on those days when you are not in the office. . . .

Making the Case for Your Proposal

Talk with other employees who have successfully negotiated flexible arrangements. Find out how they presented their proposals and use this information as you get ready to make your case. Find out about the negative experiences as well. If you want to try something that hasn't worked well before, you will [need] a viable plan for how you will deal with the obstacles or problems that have arisen in the past.

Find a flexibility "champion" or "champions" in your organization who will support you. At best, these are opinion-leaders who can either advise you behind the scenes in achieving your goal or who can take a more public stance in favor of your proposal.

Make a "business case" for greater workplace flexibility. A business case is defined as an argument where the benefits are seen as outweighing the costs:

— What is your argument? What business problem are you addressing with your request? In what ways do the benefits of your proposal outweigh any perceived problems? Why is it in your employer's self-interest to provide this flexibility?

— What is the best way to approach your supervisor? Will he or she understand this issue from firsthand experience or not? Does your supervisor respond better to a written proposal using hard data about the benefits of flexible work options for employers and employees? If so, you may want to draw on FWI [Families at Work Institute] resources to help make your case. Or does your supervisor prefer to discuss issues more informally and in person? Use the approach that best suits your supervisor's style.

— How can you best present the options for meeting your job responsibilities? Does your supervisor want to be in on the decision-making process or does he or she want you to come up with alternatives and then recommend a solution?

— How and when will the success of this arrangement be evaluated? Suggest a trial period and agree on the criteria for evaluating whether the arrangement is working or not. If problems arise, you can make changes to the arrangement. Agree to a specific timeframe when the arrangement will be evaluated and build in a process for continuing to make improvements.

If your employer does not agree to your initial proposal, would another type of flexibility work better?[67]

Be open to alternative arrangements and remain flexible. Think about how you will connect with your team so that you can collaborate and be creative. It may take some time, but creating a win-win flexible work arrangement can be the key to helping you effectively navigate work and new parenthood.

Working Families Flexibility Act of 2012

Representative Carolyn Maloney introduced legislation in 2012 called the Working Families Flexibility Act.[68] If it passes, this law would allow you to request from your employer a temporary or permanent change at work related to scheduling, number of hours worked, where work has to take place, and how far in advance you get your schedule. For example, you could ask to work part-time, ask to work from home one day per week, or ask that you get your schedule at least one month in advance so that you can make child care arrangements. Your employer would then have to hold a meeting to discuss your request and give you a decision in writing, including, if your request is rejected, the grounds for that decision (such as the cost to the business). Your employer would not be allowed to discipline or fire you just for making a request. This process is helpful not only because it would encourage workers to make requests without fear of retaliation at work, but also because many employers who are forced to explain why they are rejecting a proposal will realize there actually is no good reason for opposing an employee's plan. Keep an eye out for this important legislation!

Hourly Workers

If you are paid by the hour, you might be wondering how these ideas affect you. Can hourly workers still have flexible work arrangements? Yes, absolutely! If you work for an hourly wage, then flexibility might include shift swapping, consistent schedules, control over overtime, part-time work, breaks when you need them, and telecommuting, among other things.[69] For many hourly workers, the need is the same as for salaried workers: control over how to complete work. If a retail worker gets a drastically different schedule every week, then it might be very difficult to obtain stable child care. A server who can't swap shifts with a coworker might be unable to respond to an emergency at home.

According to research, *half* of hourly, low-wage employees work nonstandard schedules.[70] Hours are often unpredictable; for example, over 20 percent of low-wage hourly workers regularly have to work overtime with little or no notice.[71] Some workers experience a reduction in hours whenever work is slow,[72] so they can't even count on a regular paycheck. Additionally, between two-thirds and three-quarters of workers in this category do not have control over when they start and end their days at work.[73] Combined with unreliable child care arrangements and spotty transportation to work, this inflexibility can easily lead to job loss.

If your employer does not have any flexibility policies in place, you can still try negotiating to have your needs met. The same principles discussed earlier in the chapter apply: you will need to make your case as strong as possible to convince your boss that this arrangement will work.[74] Flexibility for hourly workers improves employee retention and recruitment and is good for a company's bottom line.[75] Just like with salaried employees, if your employer wants to keep a valued employee like you, they might need to be less rigid in their practices. For example, if you work for a chain, and your particular location can't find enough hours for you, ask if you can work at another location to supplement your income.[76] Finally, if you do obtain a flexible arrangement, make sure that your employer is still following the law in terms of giving you any overtime that you deserve.

Barriers to Flexibility

In an ideal world, employees would feel free to discuss their need for flexibility with their employers. Unfortunately, we know that's not the case. Many workers still fear that seeking a flexible work arrangement will have some negative impact on their career. Joan Williams, in her book *Reshaping the Work/Family Debate*, explains that flexibility is often "shelf paper" for good public relations, but few workers take advantage of existing policies (even for a short period of time) because they fear career penalties.[77] Although Williams is right—research reveals that workers who request flexibility experience negative consequences or a "flexibility stigma"—you shouldn't lose hope. There are many progressive companies that are intentional about creating a flexible work culture and that recognize workplace flexibility as a win-win. They promote an environment where workers on flexible schedules feel supported and rewarded. They know that employees who feel they can take advantage of flexible work options without penalty will be more loyal and productive workers. Even government agencies can successfully implement flexible workplace policies that focus on results and not just employee activity. A unit in a county human services and public health department in Minnesota cut case-processing times in half after implementing such a program.[78]

If you don't work for one of these leading companies with best practices, you may find yourself coming up against discrimination and stigma in your effort to manage work and family. Our next and final chapter addresses this problem and talks about a few ways in which existing law might be able to help.

As you can tell, returning to work might not be a cakewalk, but you managed to carry around a baby for nine months or make your way through the complex adoption process, so you can do this too! Remember that even though you might not have the law on your side, you can always try to convince your boss that flexibility and continued employment would benefit you both. Sometimes it just takes one brave voice to improve an employer's policies.

TOP FIVE THINGS TO REMEMBER

- You may be eligible for more time off from work after giving birth if your childbirth and postpartum recovery involved serious medical complications.
- You may be entitled to break time for pumping breast milk at work under either federal law or your state's law.
- Although no federal law generally requires your employer to provide you with a flexible work schedule at your request, you may be able to get such a schedule in certain situations covered by the Family and Medical Leave Act and the Americans with Disabilities Act.
- Check your state and local laws, as well as your employee handbook, to see whether you may be able to access paid sick time to care for your sick child and bring her or him to see the doctor.
- There may not be a law for that, but there's certainly a world of resources! Be sure to review the list of resources for this chapter for helpful tips and advice on working flexibly and finding quality child care.

4 THE PARENT TRAP
Confronting Stigma and Bias at Work

• POP QUIZ •

True or False?

1. **An employer can have a policy of hiring only employees without children and can fire anyone once he or she becomes a parent.**
   Maybe true. There is no federal law prohibiting discrimination based on someone's status as a parent. However, if an employer applies this rule only to men or just to women, it may be engaging in illegal sex discrimination.

2. **There is no legal protection for a man who faces discrimination at work because of his need to care for his husband's mother, who suffers from dementia.**
   False. Although the FMLA does not cover care for parents-in-law and doesn't recognize same-sex marriages, the ADA does protect workers from discrimination based on their need to care for a relative with a disability.

3. **Men can't sue their employers for discrimination based on caregiving because fathers are advantaged, compared to mothers, in the workplace.**
   False. Fathers also may be subject to illegal bias when they are discouraged from engaging in caregiving and expected to prioritize work above family.

Lena worked more than a decade for the same employer, where she routinely received positive reviews and was promoted multiple times. She got pregnant and took a maternity leave without any real problems, returning to work a few months after giving birth. The tone at work changed about a year later, however, when she announced that she was pregnant again. Suddenly Lena started receiving negative reviews and faced assumptions from her boss that she would not put her job first anymore. Less than two months after delivering her baby, Lena returned to work only to be told she was not capable of doing her job anymore because she was a mother. Within a few weeks she was fired.

Lena's story is real, shocking, and unfortunately, all too common. In fact, one of the fastest-growing areas of employment discrimination in America involves unfair treatment of workers because of their family responsibilities: claims of such discrimination rose nearly 400 percent in the decade between 2000 and 2010.[79] Mothers, fathers, and workers who care for their elderly and disabled loved ones are all possible targets. We hope you never have to confront such discrimination, but now that you are a parent, you may find yourself, at some point, facing bias or unfair treatment at work because of your new role. In this chapter, we want to prepare you to identify treatment that may be illegal and learn how to advocate for yourself if this should happen to you.

Before we dig into the law, we want to take you back for a moment to that "model" 1950s' family we talked about in the introduction of this book. Remember the dad heading off to work, leaving his wife to take care of the kids and the home? Well, that bygone family forms the basis for a lot of outdated assumptions about the "proper" role of mothers and fathers in the United States. Even though women now make up half of the workforce, and men increasingly take on more child care responsibilities, many employers still assume their employees will conform to the "breadwinner" and "homemaker" gender stereotypes of the past. In fact, many workplace policies on hours, pay, benefits, and leave time are designed around a male breadwinner. Modern families who try to squeeze into the existing model are like a square peg trying to fit into a round hole. But it's not *their* fault they don't fit. The problem is bigger and broader than anything an individual family can solve by itself.

One possible solution involves using discrimination laws to change the way workplaces operate and to break down outdated assumptions about parenting. But there is a slight hitch; no federal law exists expressly to protect parents from workplace discrimination. Unlike race, religion, and age, which are protected categories under the law, there is no federal law that prohibits discrimination against parents. An employer can refuse to hire parents of young children and not violate the law. In an ideal world, we would get Congress to change that. But given the glacial pace of lawmaking these days, we're not holding our breath. So for now, we have to make do with what we've got.

Luckily, advocates have been able to help parents who face bias at work using laws that prohibit discrimination based on sex, gender, pregnancy, and disability. We're going to review a couple of different situations where you or your partner might run into unfair treatment at work because of your parenting responsibilities and look at how the law might be able to help you.

Caregiver Discrimination in a Nutshell

WHAT?

Caregiver discrimination occurs when an employee (or job applicant) is unfairly penalized at work because of his or her obligation to provide care for family members. Often the discrimination grows out of stereotypes about parents and other caregivers being less committed or less capable employees. Unfair treatment can come in many forms, including being fired or not hired, being passed over for promotion, getting underpaid, having your work hours and responsibilities reduced, or being denied benefits. Harassment is also a form of discrimination, if it is severe enough and extensive enough to create a hostile work environment.

WHO?

Both men and women and both parents and childless workers can be victims of caregiver discrimination. Fathers can face discrimination for being active caregivers, when employers expect them to be dedicated to work above all else. Parents of children with disabilities may encounter bias from employers who assume they will be costly employees because of the time and resources required to care for their children. Adult children caring for aging parents may face stigma because of their caring priorities. Bottom line–anyone who needs to provide care for a loved one is vulnerable to workplace discrimination, and this means basically everyone at some point in his or her life!

WHEN?

Caregiver discrimination can impact individuals at different points in their careers and in their lives. One person might even encounter discrimination at multiple stages—for example, when pregnant, when returning to work with small children, and/or when caring for an aging parent.

WHY?

The majority of American workers are caring for a child or other relative in addition to working for pay. But many employers have not adjusted to this reality. Advocates are using antidiscrimination laws to try to change employers' assumptions and expectations about workers in today's economy and to help those workers with family responsibilities to stay employed and advance in the workplace.

MATERNAL PROFILING

Motherhood may be the most important job in the world, but plenty of bosses don't think of it that way. Many employers don't even realize that prejudice against moms can be illegal, so they say some pretty outrageous things without worrying about the consequences. Here are a few examples from real cases that made it to court in recent years:

> **A school psychologist was denied tenure after becoming a mother, despite her history of outstanding performance reviews. Her supervisors said they "did not know how [she] could perform [her] job with little ones" and thought it was "not possible for [her] to be a good mother and have this job."**

> **An executive assistant at a large bank was terminated while on maternity leave and was told by her boss,**

"When you get that baby in your arms, you're not going to want . . . to come back to work full-time . . . when a woman has a baby and she comes back to work, she's less committed to her job because she doesn't want to really be here; she wants to be with her baby."

The stereotypes that lie behind these kinds of comments—about what it means to be a good mother and a good worker—are so deeply ingrained that many employers don't even realize that what they are saying is wrong or that it could be illegal. Many employers understand that antidiscrimination laws prohibit generalizations about women as a group and the kind of blatant bias against women that was so common in the 1950s and 1960s. No longer can employers post separate job listings for men and women in the newspaper or refuse to promote a woman because she can't do "a man's job." But fewer employers understand that bias against women with children can also constitute unlawful sex discrimination, even if an employer treats childless women the same as their male peers. And under federal law (Title VII of the Civil Rights Act of 1964) and many state and local laws, gender-based stereotypes, including those about motherhood, can be evidence of such unlawful sex discrimination.

Stereotypes about mothers can crop up in dozens of ways. Below are some key triggers that may indicate unlawful discrimination. Do any of these scenarios sound familiar to you?

1. ***"Moms are just not as competent."*** You worked for your employer for years before getting pregnant and were always an excellent employee. Upon your return from childbirth, suddenly your performance reviews are no longer glowing. Your boss is hypercritical and seems to find fault in you,

but not in others who are no better at their jobs. It feels like your boss is assuming that you are less competent now that you are a mother and like your future at this job is in danger.

2. ***"Mothers are not committed to work."*** You have a one-year-old and have been back at work for months. You learn about a promotion that would mean more responsibility and also more money for you and your family. You ask your boss about the opportunity, and she says she hadn't considered you for the position because she assumed that, with a young child at home, you would not be interested in taking on more work or the travel required.
3. ***"Moms are a liability."*** You work in an office with several other women who are expecting a baby or who recently gave birth. When you announce your pregnancy to your boss, he says, "Not again! What the heck's in the water around here? I'm going to have to start hiring only guys from now on."
4. ***"Wouldn't you rather be home with your baby?"*** You return to work after delivering your baby to find that your workload and hours have been dramatically reduced. When you ask your supervisor about it, she says she decided to reallocate some of your duties while you were out on maternity leave. She adds, "It's really for the best, because this way you can spend more time with your little one."
5. ***"Moms are not as reliable."*** You are the only person in your office with kids, and you've noticed that you are also the only person whom your boss micromanages. Your boss tends to give your colleagues the benefit of the doubt whenever something goes wrong but subjects you to much stricter standards.

6. ***"It must be because she's a mom."*** You have two small kids under the age of five and have been working hard to impress your new boss. Lately, you've noticed that if you are late to a meeting by a few minutes, or you miss a detail in your work, your boss assumes your children and your family obligations are to blame, even when they are not.
7. ***"You can't do this job well and be a mother."*** You started a new job after your baby was born, to support your family, and in your first week your boss says you'll have to work until midnight. But your five-month-old daughter is in day care, and there's no one else to pick her up at the end of the day. You tell your boss about the conflict, and she tells you that it's your problem to deal with. She advises you to go home and think about whether you really want this job and suggests that maybe you think about staying home with your baby instead.
8. ***"Two's a crowd."*** You've worked with the same employer for years and didn't encounter any problems when your first child was born. When you announced your pregnancy, however, your boss guffawed and said, "Again? You do know that there are ways to prevent this from happening?" He also started making comments about how it will be easier for you to stay home with the kids once the baby is born.

These are just some of the scenarios where stereotypes about motherhood arise in the workplace. Although any one of these comments or set of facts alone might not be enough to prove discrimination, they could hint at a larger problem. If you sense that you are being treated differently than your childless coworkers or worse than you were treated before you had children, and it's threatening your job, you may want to consult an attorney or other advocate about your options.

Many women also encounter maternal profiling before they even get into a job. A recent study showed that employers are twice as likely to invite a childless woman, versus a mom, to interview for a position, whereas fathers experienced no interview callback penalty at all.[80] And what if you do get an interview but then face questions about your family? Here's a typical scene:

> Sylvia is interviewing for a job as a physician's assistant. She used to work full-time for a private medical practice but was laid off after her daughter, Elena, was born. Elena is now eighteen months old, and Sylvia is eager to return to the workforce. Her interviewer reviews her résumé and notices a gap with no work history for the past year and a half.

INTERVIEWER: So, I see that your last job ended about a year and a half ago. Have you been working since then? Or what have you been doing?

SYLVIA: Well, mostly I've been caring for my daughter, Elena.

INTERVIEWER: So you've been a stay-at-home mom? That must be nice. How old is Elena?

SYLVIA: Elena is eighteen months now. It's been great to share this amazing time with her and watch her grow, but I've also been actively keeping an eye on the job market. I am eager to jump back into work, and this position seems like the perfect opportunity, given my skills and experience.

INTERVIEWER: Who is going to take care of Elena when you go back to work? Won't that be hard for you? Would you rather just stay home?

SYLVIA: I have planned ahead for child care so that Elena will be in good hands and I will be able to dedicate myself fully to my job. As I mentioned, I am eager to get back into the medical world and use my skills to help people who need care. I think it will be good for Elena too, to see me as a working mom. I want to set an example for her.

INTERVIEWER: And you said Elena is eighteen months old? Any plans for a second child?

SYLVIA: I am really focused on my career at this time and eager to get back into patient care. I hope that I will be able to serve the patients here at Mercy Hospital and am excited to get started.

Stereotyping such as this, whether it happens in an interview or on the job, is unlawful because it shows an employer is basing his or her decision *not* on an individual woman's capabilities and performance, but on an assumption about her *because* she is a mother. Our discrimination laws are founded on the idea that people should be judged on their merits and not on their membership in a particular (and potentially disfavored) group. As one court put it, "the essence of employment discrimination is penalizing a worker not for something she did but for something she simply is . . . Women have the right to prove their mettle in the work arena without the burden of stereotypes regarding whether they can fulfill their responsibilities."[81] If your employer assumes that you will be an unreliable, unproductive, or uncommitted employee because you are a mother, when you are quite the opposite and have evidence to prove it, you may be looking at illegal stereotyping.

Although it's important to know what behavior is illegal, keep in mind that there are limits to what the law can do. It may not protect a mother who is genuinely unable to meet the expectations of her job because of her family responsibilities. In other words, if the assumption underlying the stereotype is correct—for example, your child care responsibilities make it impossible for you to work the hours regularly required by the job—then there's not much that the law can do for you. Here's one example:

> **Tasha is a single mom with a twelve-year-old daughter. She worked for her employer for over fifteen years in a full-time position with a nine-to-five schedule. When the employer eliminated Tasha's department, her boss offered her a different job requiring evening and weekend hours. Tasha was willing to work some evenings and weekends but needed those times scheduled in advance, so that she could line up someone to watch her daughter. Her employer insisted that Tasha be available for unpredictable evening hours and would not budge. Tasha was ultimately fired–her termination papers stated that "child care" was the reason for her firing.**

Federal law also does not protect a mother from bias based on her status as a parent if her employer treats men with children the same way or if the unfair treatment cannot be connected to her gender. Because the law prohibits discrimination based on sex but not based on parenthood, employers who treat fathers and mothers equally poorly are unlikely to violate the law. This is one area, like others discussed in earlier chapters, where state and local governments have done much better. Depending on where you live, the law may offer more protection, even if your employer treats both fathers and mothers poorly compared to other workers. In Alaska, for example, employment discrimination based on parenthood is illegal, and in the District of Columbia, employers are prohibited from discriminating on the basis of an employee's family responsibilities. There are also dozens of cities and counties that have similar laws.[82] Check out our state-by-state guide for more information.

Extreme Jobs and the Mommy Track:
"Attorneys without a stay-at-home spouse need not apply"

Some scholars have even argued that unlawful sex discrimination exists simply in the way workplaces and jobs, including the best-paying ones, are often built around a male breadwinner's life pattern.[83] For example, big corporate law firms often require attorneys to work through the night and sleep in the office for days. This extreme workplace assumes and expects that employees have no personal demands on their time and can dedicate 110 percent to the job. Putting aside the silliness of this assumption in general (who doesn't have some personal needs away from work, like sleeping?), it is especially problematic for women, who rarely have a spouse or partner taking care of the home front full-time. Women still shoulder much of the domestic work in today's families, and jobs that are built without any flexibility to accommodate that reality more often than not exclude women. Shunting women onto a separate "mommy track" that involves lower pay, worse hours or assignments, and little or no opportunity for advancement is no solution to the problem. Is it any wonder that women make up only 17 percent of the leadership in the nation's major law firms?

Here's one female attorney's story:

> **On my second day at [my] new firm, I was told I would be working until midnight. I explained that this was not pos-**

sible since I have an infant daughter and had to pick her up from child care. I reminded this employer that when I had accepted their offer, I had informed them that I am a new mom to a little one. I was told that this was my issue to deal with and to go home and consider whether I really wanted to be an attorney. I was also told perhaps I should return to the Midwest (where I grew up) or think about staying at home. Days later, after I had handed in my resignation, the employer relented and told me I could leave at five. However, I would be required to log back in after I had picked my daughter up and would also have to work weekends. When I would nurse my baby, spend quality time with her, etc., was irrelevant. Needless to say, I did not return to this firm. The hours would be brutal, and it was apparent that my five o'clock departure would generate great resentment. Five o'clock would turn to six, would turn to seven, and soon, I would again be sleeping under my desk like I did at my last law firm. Having to leave the firm has placed my family in dire financial straits since I was the breadwinner.

MAD MEN: DISCRIMINATION AGAINST FATHERS

We've talked about how workplaces are built to advantage male breadwinners and how this can harm mothers. But fathers also suffer at the hands of old-fashioned employers and outdated workplace policies. More fathers today want to spend time caring for children and helping to manage the home front. Many have partnered with women or men who have their own careers and are not willing to give those careers up when children enter the picture. Considering as well that many families rely on two incomes to get by, it makes sense that fathers are taking on increased responsibilities at home.

The problem arises because these new age, engaged dads buck the stereotype of a full-time breadwinner. Employers expect men to prioritize work and may even give a fatherhood bonus to men who continue to prioritize work after starting a family. They may even see dads as more stable and warmer than childless men and may reason that men with kids *need* to earn more, since they are supporting a family. But once fathers actually start doing any fatherly activities, such as asking to leave work early to pick up a sick child, the picture changes. Many dads encounter resistance from their bosses when they seek time for family. We recently surveyed over 260 dads and found that more than 12 percent of them had been penalized or had their commitment questioned when they needed to meet family responsibilities:[84]

> **"I have been questioned about my priorities."**
>
> **—attorney and father of two children, a newborn and age two**

> **"After the birth of my daughter, work kept harassing me to come back."**
>
> **—teacher and father of one child, age four**

> **"I have worked in high-pressure jobs and had a second child with serious medical issues. My spouse has a high-responsibility job as well. It was thus impossible to take adequate care of my second child and not feel like it threatened the perceptions of me in the workplace."**
>
> **—marketing consultant and father of two children, ages six and eight**

Fathers often encounter stereotypes that they cannot or should not be caregivers. In another example from our survey, one father told us,

> **"I divide child care pickup/dropoff with my wife, on a more or less 50/50 basis, and take a near equal proportion of unexpected day care closures or sick days–but I have been asked (by my CEO and board and directors), 'Why doesn't your wife [a high-level, full-time professional] care for your son in these instances?'–as if 50/50 on my end is too high a ratio."**
>
> **–nonprofit professional and father of one child, age two**

As the Supreme Court stated in 2003, "stereotypes about women's domestic roles are reinforced by parallel stereotypes presuming a lack of domestic responsibilities for men." Like the stereotypes about mothers, biased assumptions about men are firmly ingrained and may result in shocking comments from employers. For example, in a successful caregiver discrimination lawsuit, a male state trooper was denied "nurturing leave" to care for his new infant and wife, who suffered complications from her pregnancy. His employer told him that there was no way he qualified as "primary caregiver" for his wife and child and said, "God made women to have babies, and unless you would have a baby, there is no way you could be the primary caregiver."[85] The trooper won his case—and over $600,000 in damages!

So what's a dad to do if he encounters stereotypes like this at work? Luckily, fathers, like mothers, may find protection from harmful stereotyping under federal law. That's because sex-role stereotypes against fathers can also be used as evidence of unlawful gender discrimination under Title VII of the Civil Rights Act. Let's consider a possible scenario:

> **Malcolm, a new father, wants to be closely involved in the care of his baby boy. Unfortunately, all the other men with kids in his office, including his boss, have taken a much less "hands-on" approach to fatherhood. When Malcolm asks for a month of paternity leave, his boss grunts disapprovingly and says he can take off one week at most, adding, "I mean, really, Malcolm, you're not the one giving birth!" After Malcolm returns from his leave, he remains involved at home and tries to leave work every day in time to get home for his son's bedtime. His boss starts making nasty remarks about Malcolm's parenting priorities and assigns special tasks to Malcolm that always keep him at work past 7:00 p.m. The boss also neglects to tell Malcolm about numerous client-development outings and then criticizes Malcolm for not being a "team player" because he doesn't attend.**

In this hypothetical, it's pretty clear that Malcolm's boss and his workplace culture do not support Malcolm's choice to be an active father. In fact, Malcolm is being punished for prioritizing family over work instead of conforming to the breadwinner ideal. Even if this treatment doesn't end in Malcolm being fired, his boss may still be creating a hostile work environment, which is illegal as a form of harassment. Many dads in Malcolm's situation might feel defeated and forced to resign, feeling they have no alternative. But if you find this story familiar or find yourself in a similar spot at some point down the road, don't give up. Consult with an attorney or another advocate to see whether your employer is violating the law, or contact your local equal employment agency. You may be able to keep your job (and your priorities!) and help to educate your employer in the process so that other dads like you are not subject to the same treatment in the future.

Finally, in addition to stereotyping, federal law prohibits unequal treatment of men and women who are similarly situated. This means that an employer generally has to treat men with children the same as women with children would be treated. For example, if an employer allows female employees with kids to come in a bit later or leave work a bit earlier to drop off or pick up their children from school, then the employer should allow male employees the same flexibility. Keep in mind, however, that the law does allow some difference of treatment when it comes to biological differences. So an employer could offer new moms four weeks of leave as pregnancy-related disability leave but not offer the same time off to new dads. But if an employer offers caregiving leave, that must be granted equally to both men and women.

If any of these scenarios sound familiar to you, see if you can find an attorney or other advocate to speak with about your options.

DISCRIMINATION BY ASSOCIATION–CHILDREN WITH DISABILITIES

If you are the parent of a child with special needs, you may have additional protections under the law. That's because the Americans with Disabilities Act (ADA), which we described earlier in the context of pregnancy, also prohibits discrimination against employees who are related to or associated with an individual with a disability. You don't have to have a disability yourself to be protected. What does that mean in practice? If you are the parent of a child with autism, for example, your boss cannot deny you plum assignments because he assumes you will have to miss a lot of work to attend to the health and educational needs of your child. Similarly, if your child is diagnosed with Hodgkin's lymphoma, your boss may not eliminate your position because she fears that you and your family will be a drain on the company's health insurance. Here's an example from a recent court case:

> **Janet worked for a bank for over ten years, receiving raises and promotions and excellent performance reviews. She got pregnant and just before going on maternity leave was assured by her boss that she should not worry about her job, which would be waiting for her when she got back. Janet gave birth to a baby with Down Syndrome and enrolled the child in her company's health care plan four days after that. Two months later, while she was still on leave, Janet's employer eliminated her position, citing necessary reorganization of management. Janet alleged that her boss fired her because of her association with her child with a disability, and the court agreed that was a possible motivation for her termination.**[86]

As always, there are some limitations to the protections of the law. First of all, in order to qualify for protection from discrimination under the ADA, your child (or whomever you are caring for) must have a qualifying disability under the law. The ADA has been pretty strict about what constitutes a disability, requiring a mental or physical impairment that substantially limits a major life activity. But recent amendments to the law have made it easier for people with temporary and less severe disorders to qualify as having a disability. So although you may not be protected from discrimination because you are caring for a child with the flu, you might be covered if your child suffers from a severe speech impediment, even if that's temporary. There's no all-inclusive list of covered conditions, but if you suspect that you are being treated unfairly because of your need to care for a child with a disabling condition, it's probably a good idea to consult with an attorney or other advocate for more advice about your particular situation.

Second, the law in this area, like the law prohibiting discrimination based on sex, is built around the idea that employees should be judged based on their actual performance, not on their identity. This means that the same limitations we discussed before apply here—that is, if you are unable to work effectively because of your caregiving responsibilities, the law can't do much to help you. Finally, as you may remember, the ADA requires employers to provide "reasonable accommodations" to employees with disabilities, but this does *not* apply to people associated with a person with a disability under the law. So even if your employer has to offer some modification of your work schedule to accommodate your own disabling condition (such as gestational diabetes), she or he does not have to accommodate your need for flexibility because you have a child with special needs. Other state and local laws, as well as the FMLA, might help you get the time you need in this situation. Review our discussion in chapter 2 about FMLA eligibility and coverage and our state-by-state guide for more information.

Spotlight On Italy

It's hard for all parents to juggle work and family without access to paid family leave or sick days, but it can be an even bigger challenge for parents of children with special needs. We're highlighting Italy as a country that has taken important steps to support working parents of children with disabilities. According to information from the U.N.'s International Labour Organization and the European Parliament, parents of children with special needs in Italy have several legal protections that help them to balance work with their additional caregiving responsibilities. Mothers and fathers of a seriously disabled child may take additional paid parental leave beyond what is available to all new parents in Italy, and may take this extra leave in one of two ways. These parents can take up to three years off–all at once or incrementally–until the child's eighth birthday at 30 percent of their normal wage. Alternatively, they may take two hours of paid break time per day until the child's third birthday, and three days off per month after their child turns three. Parents of children with special needs also have the right to choose a place of work closer to home, and cannot be transferred to another location without their consent.

Even for children without special needs, parents in Italy are entitled to stay home from work to care for an ill child under three. For foster and adoptive parents, this period extends until the child is six. After this period ends, parents are still able to take up to five paid days off per year to care for a biological child age three to eight, or an adoptive or foster child age six to twelve.

Eldercare

Eldercare is not the focus of this book, but as the sandwich generation, we know a large percentage of you are taking care of little ones and parents or other elderly relatives. There are some legal protections for those of you providing eldercare too.

First, the ADA's prohibition against associational discrimination, discussed previously, also applies to an adult who has a parent or another relative with a disability. For example, an employer who assumes his employee will be too distracted by her grandfather's Alzheimer's disease to be productive and demotes her as a result could very well be violating the law.

Second, the Family and Medical Leave Act (FMLA; see chapter 2) guarantees eligible workers time to care for a family member suffering from a "serious medical condition." For example, if a worker needs time off to take her mother to chemotherapy appointments, she could probably take that time under the FMLA and would be protected from retaliation for doing so. Unfortunately, a worker would not be able to do the same for her mother-in-law because only parents (and those who parented the employee when she was under eighteen) are covered under the law. However, some states have expanded the group of family members who may be cared for using family leave, so check our state-by-state guide for more details about your home state.

UNFAIR TREATMENT: EQUAL PAY AND OTHER BENEFITS

You've probably heard the statistic that women make only seventy-seven cents for every dollar a man earns. This pay gap exists despite the fact that it's been illegal to pay men and women unequal wages for the same work for fifty years! In a majority of jobs across the economy, women still earn less than their male counterparts.[87] And mothers suffer additional pay penalties: they earn about 5 percent less per child than their childless female peers.[88] That means that a mother of three earns *15 percent* less than her childless counterpart.

Contrary to what some skeptics say, the pay gap cannot be explained by women's choices—for example, to work part-time, to seek jobs that offer more flexibility, and so on. Even accounting for differences in education, experience, and time out of the workforce, over 40 percent of the wage gap remains unexplained, which really means discrimination is to blame.[89] Pregnancy discrimination and maternal profiling, which push women into lower-paying jobs or out of the workplace altogether, certainly contribute to women's lifetime earnings loss. Scientists have also tested for maternal wage discrimination in hiring and found it alive and well. In one study, participants were asked to evaluate pairs of résumés and say how likely they would be to hire each person and how much they would pay them.[90] The trick? The résumés were identical except that one woman stated her leadership role in the PTA, and the other woman had a neighborhood association on her résumé instead. The study also tested fathers and childless men. The result? Participants in the study were more likely to hire childless women, childless men, and fathers than mothers, and they offered mothers $11,000 less per year in pay, on average, than equally qualified childless candidates.[91]

So what's a mother to do? First, in order to protect yourself from discrimination, you need to know what the law provides. Two federal laws outlaw discrimination on the basis of sex in the payment of wages or benefits: Title VII of the Civil Rights Act of 1964 (Title VII) broadly prohibits sex discrimination in compensation, whereas the Equal Pay Act of 1963 (EPA) prohibits employers from paying men and women in the same workplace unequal wages for equal work. Both laws cover all forms of compensation, including salary, overtime pay, bonuses, vacation, and other benefits. Although the EPA covers more people than Title VII, which applies only to employers with fifteen or more employees, it's generally harder to use because it requires comparison between you and someone else doing equal (rather than substantially similar) work.

The Equal Pay Act of 1963 in a Nutshell

WHAT?

The Equal Pay Act (EPA) requires equal pay for equal work performed under similar working conditions in the same establishment. This means that employers have to pay men and women doing the same jobs equally. However, if salaries are based on any factor other than sex, such as a seniority system, a merit system, or a system that measures earnings by quantity or quality of production, there is no violation of the law.

WHO?

This law applies to any employer with two or more employees. The law does apply to both full-time and part-time workers, but comparisons generally can't be made between part-time and full-time workers at an establishment. In other words, if a female part-time worker is making less than a full-time male coworker, then she probably won't be able to use this law, since part-time status is considered a factor other than sex.

HOW?

Two jobs are equal when they require equal levels of skill, effort, and responsibility and are performed under similar conditions. The focus is on the duties performed. Job titles, classifications, and descriptions may factor in but do not, by themselves, determine the answer.

WHEN?

If you believe you are being paid less because of your sex, you have two years to file with the EEOC or go directly to court. If you also would like to file a charge under Title VII (for sex discrimination), then you have 180 days to file a charge with the EEOC. Federal employees have forty-five days to contact an Equal Employment Office counselor.[92]

WHY?

When the EPA was passed, women were taking home just fifty-nine cents for every dollar a man earned. That pay gap has narrowed over time but still persists. Congress and some states are considering laws to amend the EPA and expand protections for working women, including prohibiting punishment of employees who share salary information with their coworkers in order to uncover wage disparities. To learn more about these and other proposals, check out our list of resources on page 183.

If you suspect unequal pay, you might want to ask around to find out what other people doing similar work are being paid. Here's one example of a woman we met through our work:

> **Carol was curious what her colleague, Jim, earned for his year-end bonus, and Jim was curious about Carol's bonus. The two decided to share their numbers with each other and discovered that Jim was paid about $5,000 more than Carol in bonus pay, even though she worked hard at the same job, coming in early and leaving late nearly every day.**

But beware! According to a 2010 study, 61 percent of private-sector employees reported that they are discouraged or prohibited from discussing wage and salary information.[93] The National Labor Relations Board has interpreted federal law to prohibit total bans on wage discussions, but the law only covers certain workers, leaving others, such as supervisory employees, without protection. Lilly Ledbetter, whose case we discussed at the end of chapter 1, is a good example. She worked as a supervisor at Goodyear Tire for nearly twenty years before an anonymous tip revealed she was being paid less than her male colleagues. Had Lilly asked her colleagues directly about their pay, the law would not have protected her from retaliation.[94] A few states have made it illegal to penalize workers for sharing salary and wage information, so definitely check our state-by-state guide to see whether you live in one of those states. If not, you may want to tread carefully before making inquiries about others' paychecks.

Finally, if you think your rights have been violated, don't hesitate to seek advice. Although you are not required to file a charge with the Equal Employment Opportunity Commission under the

EPA, you are required to do so under Title VII. Thanks to the Lilly Ledbetter Fair Pay Act, you now have at least 180 days from the time you receive a discriminatory pay check (maybe more, depending on your home state) to file a charge of discrimination under Title VII.

The Part-Time Penalty

Many mothers, and some fathers, work part-time in order to balance their work and family responsibilities. Still others work part-time because they cannot find full-time work. Not only do these workers earn less by virtue of working fewer hours, but they are also paid on average about 20 percent less per hour than full-time workers doing the same or similar work. Part-time workers are also far less likely than their full-time colleagues to have access to benefits such as paid sick days, health insurance, or retirement benefits.

Unfortunately, current law does little to prevent this kind of unfair treatment. Some of our laws explicitly exclude part-time workers from protection. For example, the FMLA, as described in chapter 2, covers only workers who have worked at least 1,250 hours in the twelve months leading up to their leave. That means that an expecting parent who has worked fewer than twenty-four hours per week throughout the year may not be able to take time off to care for a new child. Plenty of parents work two or more part-time jobs to keep their family afloat, and many others simply cannot find full-time employment. Do these parents and their children deserve so much less than full-time workers and their families?

This is just one of the many areas where the United States can do better. In Europe, policies aimed at improving part-time work are widespread, thanks largely to a 1997 EU Directive on Part-Time Work, whose official purpose was "to eliminate discrimination against part-time workers and to improve the quality of part-time work."

We hope this chapter has helped to expand your understanding of what is legal and what's not when it comes to discrimination against parents in the workplace. Being wise in the ways of the law can help you to stand up for yourself when you suspect unfair treatment.

TOP FIVE THINGS TO REMEMBER

- Your employer's assumption that you'd rather spend more time with your kids, just because you are a mom, even if based on good intentions, is still evidence of unlawful discrimination.
- Dads—not just moms—can also be victims of discrimination on the job and may seek protection under federal law.
- Although your boss may not penalize you for having a child with disabilities, she or he is not required to alter the job to help you manage your child's care.
- If you suspect you are being paid less because of gender-based discrimination, you have at least 180 days from each bias-tainted paycheck to file a charge of discrimination with the Equal Employment Opportunity Commission.
- You may be able to resolve your workplace conflict without going to court. Putting your suspicions in writing to a human resources manager or other superior can put your employer on notice that you are savvy about your rights and may convince them to change their ways.

CONCLUSION

Pregnancy and parenthood can be intimidating. The physical and emotional changes that come with this stage of life are more than enough to leave you reeling. But imagine facing discrimination or other problems at work while also trying to manage your new family reality. The combination can be devastating to your health and happiness, not to mention your bank account.

As lawyers, we encounter too many people who simply aren't aware of their rights. We talk with expecting and new parents every week (you've read some of their stories in this book) who don't realize the potential of existing laws, which can protect them from unfair treatment or offer some help in the struggle to balance work and family. Ignorance is a powerful barrier to justice. What good is a law if people don't know about it and are unable to benefit from its protections?

As advocates, our first priority is helping you and other working parents understand the rights you *do* have. That's a major part of why we wrote this book! We want to empower you to speak up for yourself or find the help you need to get what you deserve. But we also recognize that there's plenty more our country could do to help families like yours. We can work to clarify and expand our existing laws to cover more people than they currently do. We can eliminate legal hurdles so that folks who are protected by the law can exercise their rights more easily. And we can push our workplace laws and policies into the twenty-first century so that they finally catch up to the way people live and work today. For many families, the need for such reform is dire. Here's one (final!) heartbreaking story from a real family, which we heard from a pediatric nurse in New York:

> **Monica and John faced an impossible choice when they learned their young daughter, Julia, was dying of cancer. Monica's eyes filled with tears, and John held Julia a little bit tighter in his arms as the nurse told them gently there was nothing else to be done to save her life. The sadness in the room was overpowering. After an explanation of what they might encounter in the next few days, the conversation took a dramatic change in direction. Could John take time off from work to spend the last few days of his little girl's life by her side? Should the doctor send a letter to his boss? John didn't want to miss a single moment with his dying daughter, so he chose to be with her and go a week without pay. A week without pay would take a serious financial toll on the family because Monica didn't earn any income, they had another child to support, and they had mounting medical bills to pay. The pediatric nurse who cared for Julia wondered, "How do you ask a parent to make a decision between supporting their family and spending what little time is left with their daughter before she dies? What then happens if a week passes and she hangs on even longer? Should a parent have to miss the last few breaths of his daughter's life because he might lose his job if he takes more time off? How can that question be asked of a grieving parent?"**

How *do* we, as a country, ask these questions of our parents? Why do we? For a nation whose politicians tout family values at every opportunity, we have done shockingly little to value the critical work of families. We can do so much better. But how do we get there? How do we make our country into one that truly values families? We need wide-ranging solutions. We have all seen the recklessness of leaving these problems to individual families to work out on their own. Here at A Better Balance we are working on a slew of ideas to support pregnant workers, guarantee family leave insurance and paid sick days, extend protections for caregivers in the workplace, and promote flexible and reliable work practices. We work at the local, state, and national levels, advocating for policies to help American workers get the time and flexibility they need to care for their families. Here are just a few examples (at the national level) of the kinds of solutions we and our partner organizations are working on:

> ***The Breastfeeding Promotion Act.*** Although the Affordable Care Act of 2010 guarantees some workers break time and a private place to express breast milk, others are still not covered. This bill would extend those rights to executive, administrative, and professional employees, including elementary and secondary school teachers, and would make clear that federal law prohibits discrimination against breastfeeding women as a form of sex discrimination.
>
> ***The Pregnant Workers Fairness Act.*** Existing law too often leaves pregnant women worse off than coworkers with similar physical limitations. This bill is designed to ensure that pregnant workers are not forced out of their jobs unnecessarily or

denied reasonable job modifications that would allow them to continue working and supporting their families.

The FAMILY Act. Too many Americans simply cannot afford to take unpaid time off to care for a new child or an ill loved one. A federal proposal, funded by minimal employer and employee contributions, would allow family caregivers to draw benefits in order to stay afloat financially when their families need them most.

The Family and Medical Leave Enhancement Act and ***The Family and Medical Leave Inclusion Act.*** Too many Americans are simply not covered by the FMLA. The first of these bills would expand coverage to employers with twenty-five or more employees and expand the reasons a worker is allowed to take leave, including parental involvement in school and routine medical needs. The second would expand the definition of "family member," making it possible for workers to use leave time to care for a domestic partner, parent-in-law, adult child, sibling, grandchild, or grandparent.

The Healthy Families Act. Forty million Americans don't have even one single paid sick day that they can use to care for themselves or a sick child. This bill would allow workers across the country to earn up to seven days per year of paid sick time to use for sickness and doctor visits and to take care of an ailing family member.

Paycheck Fairness Act. Nearly fifty years after the Equal Pay Act became law, women still earn only seventy-seven cents for every dollar men earn. This bill would strengthen the Equal Pay Act to make it more effective, improving remedies for pay discrimination and prohibiting employers from retaliating against workers who share salary information, among other things.

Working Families Flexibility Act of 2012. A majority of working Americans wish they had more flexibility and predictability in their work schedules, but they fear the negative consequences of asking for it. This bill would guarantee workers the right to request an alternative work schedule and would require employers to consider such requests formally, while prohibiting retaliation against employees for making such a request. Note that this is different from the Working Families Flexibility Act of 2013, which is about compensatory time.

For more information about our work and updates on our latest campaigns, please visit our website at www.abetterbalance.org. You can also follow us on social media at www.twitter.com/abetterbalance and www.facebook.com/abetterbalance.

We've told you what we're doing, but what can you do? Lots! Even with just a few minutes of your time, you can help immeasurably to push this cause forward. We've given you a head start: we've brainstormed ideas for how to change the laws, we've helped to write new laws, and we've done lots of research to support them. But we need to hear from you! We need you, your family, and your friends to speak up and let your representatives know that these issues are important to you and that you will vote for politicians who prioritize them. If elected officials hear only from advocates like us and not from their constituents, they are unlikely to put the needs of working families at the top of their to-do lists. In politics, money and the masses hold the most influence. We need you—and the power of your extended networks—to start a movement.

TAKE ACTION!

Here's a list of the top five things you can do right now to change the way America works:

Speak Up! Call, write, email, or visit your elected officials and ask them what they are doing to improve workplace laws for families. If they are not supporting proposed legislation on this issue, ask them why. Not sure who your representatives are? You can search for your congressional representatives and your state and local officials by zip code or by address online.

Keep Informed! Our website is a great place to start for information about the work–family crunch and policies proposed to address it. You can also learn about our partner organizations and what they are doing to further the cause and can find links to the latest research and news about what's happening now.

Start a Conversation! Use this book to open a dialogue with friends about how the work–family crunch has impacted them and engage them in this movement. Maybe even start a book club, or if you're already a member, suggest this book for discussion.

Share Your Story! As you've seen throughout this book, real stories are incredibly powerful tools for informing and moving people to action. If you feel comfortable sharing your experiences, anonymously or not, please let us know by emailing babygate@abetterbalance.org. We would love to hear from you.

Volunteer! If you've gotten fired up and are looking for more to do, there are lots of great organizations around the country working on these issues that could use your time or donations. Check out our partners' links on our website and do some Internet searches to find out which groups are in your neck of the woods.

We have covered a lot of information in this book, and we don't blame you if you are feeling overwhelmed. But we truly believe that knowledge is power: the more you know, the more you can advocate for yourself in the workplace. We stand behind you every step of the way. Good luck in your journey through pregnancy and parenthood! And we hope that despite the frenzy and fatigue of your new role, you will still feel inspired to join us in bringing a better balance to all Americans.

RESOURCES

CHAPTER 1

For more information about unemployment insurance and pregnancy/family responsibilities, check out the National Employment Law Project's report *Between a Rock and a Hard Place: Confronting the Failure of State Unemployment Insurance Systems to Serve Women and Working Families* at http://nelp.3cdn.net/ebba1e75e059fc749d_0um6idptk.pdf.

For more information about pregnancy in the workplace check out the National Women's Law Center (www.nwlc.org), the National Partnership for Women and Families (www.nationalpartnership.org), and the ACLU Women's Rights Project (www.aclu.org/womens-rights).

For other legal issues that may impact you as a pregnant woman, check out Legal Momentum at www.legalmomentum.org and National Advocates for Pregnant Women at http://advocatesforpregnantwomen.org.

To better understand the rights of childbearing women, view this brochure: http://www.childbirthconnection.org/pdfs/rights_childbearing_women.pdf and visit www.childbirthconnection.org.

If you are looking for more information about possible accommodations for pregnancy-related limitations, visit the Job Accommodation Network (JAN) at http://askjan.org.

For information on how to file a charge of pregnancy discrimination, check out the Equal Employment Opportunity Commission's website: http://www.eeoc.gov/employees/howtofile.cfm.

If you are looking for a lawyer to represent you, the National Employment Lawyers Association has a search tool on its website at http://www.nela.org/NELA/.

Pregnancy-Related Complications and Accommodations That Could Qualify for Americans with Disabilities Act (ADA) Coverage

This list, from our partners at WorkLife Law, includes many complications and medical issues that women experience during pregnancy. Each heading is a medical issue that you might face, followed by example accommodations you might need in the workplace. If you have one of these medical conditions, then you may qualify for coverage under ADA or local disability laws. See page 41 or speak to an attorney for more information.

ABNORMAL BLEEDING

Time off for medical appointments

Scheduling changes such as telework (which may include a transfer to a position that provides this kind of flexibility)

Lifting assistance or limitations

Using assistive equipment to lift

Modification of the duties of the job, such as temporary light duty

Move workstation close to restrooms

BACK PAIN (LUMBAR LORDOSIS)
Use of a heating pad
Sitting instead of standing
Lifting assistance or limitations
Using assistive equipment to lift
Modification of the duties of the job, such as temporary light duty

BLOOD CLOT
Time off for medical appointments
Modification of work station to allow elevation of legs
Short breaks for movement or exercise

CARPAL TUNNEL SYNDROME
Occasional breaks from manual tasks or typing and specialized programs that allow for dictation instead of typing
Ergonomic support for hands and wrists

CHRONIC MIGRAINES
Changing lighting in the work area
Limiting exposure to noise and fragrances
Scheduling changes such as flexible schedules or telework (which may include a transfer to a position that provides this kind of flexibility)

DEPENDENT EDEMA
Provide employee with stool or chair to sit on while working
Modification of work station to allow elevation of legs
Short breaks for movement or exercise
Modification of footwear requirements

DYSPNEA (SHORTNESS OF BREATH)
Provide employee with stool or chair to sit on while working
Using assistive equipment to lift
Modification of the duties of the job, such as temporary light duty

FATIGUE
Light duty to avoid strenuous activity
Flexible or reduced hours
Exemption from mandatory overtime

GASTROESOPHAGEAL REFLUX (GERD)
Allowing for breaks for food as needed
Providing space for medications to be stored

GESTATIONAL DIABETES
Time off for medical appointments
Permission to take more frequent bathroom breaks and to eat small snacks during work hours
Breaks and a private location for testing blood glucose
Provide space for medications to be stored
Scheduling changes such as flexible schedules or telework (which may include a transfer to a position that provides this kind of flexibility)

HEMORRHOIDS
Allow women to avoid being in a seated position all day or to use a special cushion

HYPEREMESIS GRAVIDARUM; "MORNING SICKNESS"
Permission to take more frequent bathroom breaks
Permission to eat small snacks during work hours
A cot for lying down
Scheduling changes such as flexible schedules or telework (which may include a transfer to a position that provides this kind of flexibility)

INTRAUTERINE GROWTH RESTRICTION
Scheduling changes such as telework (which may include a transfer to a position that provides this kind of flexibility)

PERINATAL DEPRESSION
Time off for employee to participate in therapeutic sessions
Temporary transfer to a less distracting environment
Telecommuting
Leave

PRETERM LABOR RISK
Time off for medical appointments
Scheduling changes such as flexible schedules or telework (which may include a transfer to a position that provides this kind of flexibility)

Lifting assistance or limitations
Using assistive equipment to lift
Modification of the duties of the job, such as temporary light duty
Move workstation close to restrooms

SYMPHYSEAL SEPARATION
Modification of work station with ability to sit or stand as needed
Scheduling changes such as telework (which may include a transfer to a position that provides this kind of flexibility)

SYNCOPE OR NEAR-SYNCOPE
Providing a stool or chair to sit on
More frequent breaks
Lifting assistance or limitations
Using assistive equipment to lift
Modification of the duties of the job, such as temporary light duty
Move workstation close to restrooms

URINARY FREQUENCY
More frequent bathroom breaks
Carrying a bottle of water

VARICOSE VEINS
Short breaks for movement or exercise
Modification of work station with ability to sit or stand as needed.

CHAPTER 2

The Department of Labor, which enforces the FMLA, has a helpful guide for employees available at http://www.dol.gov/whd/fmla/employeeguide.htm.

To get a sense of what other employers may provide in terms of parental leave, and for other research on family-friendly workplaces, check out the Families and Work Institute at http://www.familiesandwork.org/.

To find out more about what unions and collective bargaining agreements may offer for parental leave, check out the Labor Project for Working Families at http://www.working-families.org/#social=twtr.

For a proposal template and a negotiation guide, along with other practical tips for getting the most out of your maternity leave, check out the Maternity Leave Mentor (Pat Katepoo) and her Max Your Maternity Leave guide at http://www.maternityleavementor.com.

For more state-by-state information about job-protected time off, check out Workplace Flexibility 2010's overview at http://workplaceflexibility2010.org/images/uploads/EXTOJobProtection.pdf.

To learn more about what your state does (or does not do) for families, check out the National Partnership for Women and Families' report *Expecting Better: A State-by-State Analysis of Laws That Help New Parents* at http://www.nationalpartnership.org/site/DocServer/Expecting_Better_Report.pdf?docID=10301.

For information on how to file a complaint with the Department of Labor about a violation of the FMLA, please visit the Wage and Hour Division website, http://www.dol.gov/whd/america2.htm, to find the contact information for your local office.

For information about military family leave, check out this FAQ fact sheet from the Department of Labor: http://www.dol.gov/whd/fmla/finalrule/MilitaryFAQs.pdf.

CHAPTER 3

Lactation/Breastfeeding at Work

Information about breastfeeding at work, for both employers and employees, is available in the Corporate Voices for Working Families Workplace Lactation Toolkit: http://www.cvworkingfamilies.org/lactation.

If you and/or your employer need help establishing a lactation-friendly workplace, check out Worksites for Wellness at http://www.worksitesforwellness.org/ for helpful tips and information.

For an employee's guide to breastfeeding and working, check out the US Department of Health and Human Services resource "The Business Case for Breastfeeding: Steps for Creating a Breastfeeding Friendly Worksite" at http://www.womenshealth.gov/breastfeeding/government-in-action/business-case-for-breastfeeding/employee%27s-guide-to-breastfeeding-and-working.pdf.

Flexible/Predictable Work Schedules

For research, news, and other resources for customizing your workplace practices, visit www.customfitworkplace.org, an initiative of MomsRising.org.

For more factual background on the benefits of workplace flexibility, see Workplace Flexibility 2010, Georgetown University Law Center, at http://workplaceflexibility2010.org/index.php/why_it_matters/.

For tips on implementing flexible workplace policies successfully, check out the Workplace Flexibility Toolkit, "When Work Works," created by the Families and Work Institute in partnership with the US Chamber of Commerce's Institute for a Competitive Workforce and the Twiga Foundation, at http://familiesandwork.org/3w/toolkit/web page-toolkit.html.

Corporate Voices for Working Families also offer toolkits on workplace flexibility, including specific toolkits for hourly workers and their managers, at http://www.cvworkingfamilies.org/publication-toolkits/tips-managers-employees.

The Maternity Leave Mentor (mentioned above in chapter 2 resources) has flexible return-to-work resources on her website at http://www.maternityleavementor.com.

National polling data is now available at the Center for American Progress, www.americanprogress.org/wp-content/uploads/issues/2010/03/pdf/work_survey.pdf, showing broad public support for public policies to address work–family conflict.

The 2008 National Study of Employers (NSE) by the Families and Work Institute, familiesandwork.org/site/research/reports/2008nse.pdf, presents workplace practices, policies, programs, and benefits in use at companies around the country.

For union workplaces, check out Flex Pack: A Toolkit on Organizing, Bargaining, and Legislating for Worker-Controlled Flexibility, at Labor Project for Working Families, http://www.working-families.org/publications/flexpack.pdf.

Working Mother magazine has research on the best companies to work for, including their review, with Flex-Time Lawyers, of the best law firms for women, http://www.flextimelawyers.com/best/p11a.pdf, and their report on best companies for hourly employees, http://www.wmmsurveys.com/2012_HW_exec_summary.pdf.

Child Care

The National Women's Law Center has many resources about child care, although most of them are geared toward policy makers, not parents. (This is the general website for that issue: http://www.nwlc.org/our-issues/child-care-%2526-early-learning.)

This report details specific state policies on child care assistance, such as income eligibility for assistance, waiting lists, and reimbursement rates: http://www.nwlc.org/sites/default/files/pdfs/state_child_care_assistance_policies_report2011_final.pdf.

To learn more about policy proposals at the national and state level that impact infants, toddlers, and their families, visit Zero to Three at http://www.zerotothree.org/public-policy.

For a report on tax credits at the state level, check out http://www.urban.org/UploadedPDF/1000796_Tax_Fact_7-11-05.pdf (but note that the report is from 2005, so just use this as a jumping-off point).

The National Association for the Education of Young Children (www.naeyc.org) has many resources for parents. Search "parents" for information on pamphlets and books about finding quality care. The website includes a page for searching for NAEYC-accredited programs: http://families.naeyc.org/find-quality-child-care.

ChildCare Aware (formerly the National Network of Child Care Resource and Referral), at www.naccrra.org, can be used for information on finding quality care: http://childcareaware.org/parents-and-guardians.

The National Child Care Information Center (NCCIC), http://www.nifa.usda.gov/nea/family/part/childcare_part_nccic.html, is a government-sponsored website offering resources and information related to child care.

The organization Child Care Resources, Inc., http://www.childcareresourcesinc.org/, can also help you learn about quality child care and search for child care.

Here is an explanation of the Child and Dependent Care Tax Credit: http://www.taxcreditsforworkingfamilies.org/child-and-dependent-care-tax-credit/.

An organization in New York City, Park Slope Parents, has a helpful website for parents who are also employers or are thinking of becoming employers. Although the group is specific to New Yorkers, there is information that can help anyone learn how to be a great employer: http://www.parkslopeparents.com/index.php?option=com_content&task=blogcategory&id=50&Itemid=185. Hand in Hand, the Domestic Employers Association, can also help: http://domesticemployers.org/.

There are also many local organizations offering support in this area, such as the Child Care Resource Center (www.ccrcinc.org) in Boston or the Center for Children's Initiatives (CCI), which provides free child care referral services to New York City parents: www.centerforchildrensinitiatives.org.

CHAPTER 4

The Center for WorkLife Law has lots of research and information about caregiver discrimination and hosts a hotline you can call if you believe you may be facing this kind of bias at work. Visit them at http://worklifelaw.org/frd.

9to5, National Association of Working Women has a Job Survival Helpline, with information and referrals about employment rights, including discrimination. You can reach them at (800) 522-0925 or by emailing them at helpline@9to5.org.

The Equal Employment Opportunity Commission issued guidance about caregiver discrimination in 2007 and followed in 2009 with Best Practices for Employers. Both documents are available online: http://www.eeoc.gov/policy/docs/caregiving.html and http://www.eeoc.gov/policy/docs/caregiver-best-practices.html.

Workforce 21C offers information tailored for employers who are trying to do the right thing and offers more background on caregiver discrimination. If you are trying to work with your employer to develop better workplace policies, you can direct them to http://www.workforce21c.com/index.html to help guide your conversation.

For more information about the wage gap and resources on how to combat it on the job, you can check out WAGE (the Women Are Getting Even Project) at http://www.wageproject.org/index.php.

NOTES

1. Eve Tahmincioglu, "Pregnancy Bias Is Alive and Well in America," *Today Show*, MSNBC, February 15, 2012, http://lifeinc.today.msnbc.msn.com/_news/2012/02/15/10417141-pregnancy-bias-is-alive-and-well-in-america?lite.
2. Sarah Jane Glynn, *The New Breadwinners: 2010 Update* (Center for American Progress, April 2012), 2.
3. Kelleen Kay and David Gray, *The Stress of Balancing Work and Family: The Impact on Parents and Child Health and the Need for Workplace Flexibility* (New America Foundation, 2007), http://www.newamerica.net/publications /policy/stress_balancing_work_and_family.
4. Eduardo Porter, "Motherhood Still a Cause of Pay Inequality," *New York Times*, June 13, 2012.
5. Jody Heymann and Alison Earle, *Raising the Global Floor: Dismantling the Myth That We Can't Afford Good Working Conditions for Everyone* (Stanford University Press, 2010), 111. The total number includes Australia, which began a national paid parental leave scheme in 2011.
6. Ibid., 143.
7. *Table 5-g, Maternity Leave Benefits* (United Nations Statistics Division, Statistics and Indicators on Men and Women, December 2011), http://unstats.un.org/unsd/demographic/products/indwm/Tables_Excel/table5g_Dec%202011.xls.
8. Katherine Marshall, *Fathers' Use of Paid Parental Leave* (Statistics Canada, Catalogue no. 75-001-X, June 2008), 8, http://www.statcan.gc.ca/pub/75-001-x/2008106/pdf/10639-eng.pdf.
9. Linda Laughlin, *Maternity Leave and Employment Patterns of First-Time Mothers: 1961–2008* (US Census Bureau, Current Population Reports, P70-128, October 2011), http://www.census.gov/prod/2011pubs/p70-128.pdf.
10. Heymann and Earle, *Raising the Global Floor*, 107.
11. *Govori v. Goat Fifty*, LLC, No. 10 Civ. 8982(DLC), 2011 WL 1197942 (S.D.N.Y. March 30, 2011).

12. See written testimony of Joan C. Williams, "Unlawful Discrimination against Pregnant Workers and Workers with Caregiving Responsibilities" (US Equal Employment Opportunity Commission, February 15, 2012), http://www.eeoc.gov/eeoc/meetings/2-15-12/williams.cfm#fn1. "Guidance is needed to clarify that if a woman's doctor orders a restriction required to protect her ability to deliver a healthy, full-term baby, she is entitled to reasonable accommodation because delivering a baby is a major bodily function and life activity under the ADAAA."
13. Childbirth Connection, a program of National Partnership for Women & Families, "Listening to Mothers: The Experiences of Expecting and New Mothers in the Workplace," January 2014, available at: http://www.nationalpartnership.org/research-library/workplace-fairness/pregnancy-discrimination/listening-to-mothers-experiences-of-expecting-and-new-mothers.pdf.
14. Other states also have laws that may allow for workplace modifications for pregnant women. Please check the state-by-state guide for more details.
15. 29 C.F.R. § 1604.10(c) (1979).
16. National Partnership for Women & Families, "A Look at the U.S. Department of Labor's 2012 Family and Medical Leave Act Employee and Worksite Surveys" (February 2013), available at: http://go.nationalpartnership.org/site/DocServer/DOL_FMLA_Survey_2012_Key_Findings.pdf?docID=1186.
17. As of 2012, implementation of Washington State's Paid Family and Medical Leave Insurance law has been postponed until October 2015.
18. A Better Balance, "Investing in Our Families: The Case for Family Leave Insurance in New York and the Nation," Sept. 2013, http://abetterbalance.org/web/images/stories/Documents/familyleave/ FLI2013.pdf.
19. Childbirth may be considered a disability under New York State law and could trigger an employer's duty to provide reasonable accommodations in the form of limited time off. The New York City Pregnant Workers Fairness Act covers time off for recovery from childbirth.
20. *Why Breastfeeding Is Important* (US Department of Health and Human Services, Office on Women's Health, August 2010), http://www.womenshealth.gov/breastfeeding/why-breastfeeding-is-important/.
21. "For Employees: How Do I Get Support for Breastfeeding When I Return to Work?" Worksites for Wellness, accessed January 10, 2013, http://www.worksitesforwellness.org/how-do-i-get-support-for-breastfeeding-when-i-return-to-work.html.
22. Ibid.
23. Adapted from *The Business Case for Breastfeeding: Steps for Creating a Breastfeeding-Friendly Worksite* (US Department of Health and Human Services, Health Resources and Services Administration [HSRA], Maternal and Child Health Bureau, 2008), http://www.womenshealth.gov/breastfeeding/government-in-action/business-case-for-breastfeeding/employee%27s-guide-to-breastfeeding-and-working.pdf.
24. *Prevalence of Self-Reported Postpartum Depressive Symptoms—17 States, 2004–2005* (Centers for Disease Control, Morbidity and Mortality Weekly Report, 57(14): 361–66, April 11, 2008), http://www.cdc.gov/MMWR/preview/mmwrhtml/mm5714a1.htm

25. Child Care Aware of America, *Parents and the High Cost of Child Care* (2012), http://www.naccrra.org.
26. *America's Report Card 2012: Children in the U.S.* (First Focus and Save the Children), 8, http://www.childrenshungeralliance.org.
27. Ibid.
28. "Childcare," Embassy of France in Washington, published July 13, 2012, accessed March 25, 2013, http://ambafrance-us.org/spip.php?article555.
29. Ibid.
30. Mary Becker, "Caring for Children and Caretakers," *Chicago-Kent Law Review* 76 (2001): 1495.
31. Claire Lundberg, "Trapped by European-style Socialism—And I Love It!," *Slate*, November 2, 2012, http://www.slate.com/articles/life/family/2012/11/socialist_child_care_in_europe_creche_ecole_maternelle_and_french_child.single.html.
32. Ibid.
33. *Child Care and Development Fund* (US Department of Health and Human Services, Office of Child Care, March 2012), 1, http://www.acf.hhs.gov/sites/default/files/occ/ccdf_factsheet.pdf.
34. Ibid.
35. Sharmila Lawrence and J. Lee Kreader, *Parent Employment and the Use of Child Care Subsidies—Research Brief* (Child Care and Early Education Research Connections, 2006), 3, http://academiccommons.columbia.edu/catalog/ac:127367.
36. Karen Schulman and Helen Blank, *State Child Care Assistance Policies 2011: Reduced Support for Families in Challenging Times* (National Women's Law Center, October 2011), 1, http://www.nwlc.org/sites/default/files/pdfs/state_child_care_assistance_policies_report2011_final.pdf.
37. *Affordability: Women and Their Families Need Help Paying for Child Care* (National Women's Law Center, February 2008), 2, http://www.nwlc.org/sites/default/files/pdfs/AffordabilityMarch2008.pdf.
38. "Topic 602—Child and Dependent Care Credit," Internal Revenue Service, last modified January 7, 2013, accessed January 11, 2013, http://www.irs.gov/taxtopics/tc602.html.
39. Ibid.
40. Ibid.
41. Elaine Maag, "State Tax Credits for Child Care," *Tax Notes* (Tax Policy Center, July 11, 2005), http://www.urban.org/UploadedPDF/1000796_Tax_Fact_7-11-05.pdf.
42. "Head Start Services," Administration for Children and Families, accessed January 11, 2013, http://transition.acf.hhs.gov/programs/ohs/about/head-start. Use this Head Start Locator to find Head Start centers near you: http://eclkc.ohs.acf.hhs.gov/hslc/HeadStartOffices. Find out about registration and whether or not you are eligible by going to "Register for the Program," Administration for Children and Families, accessed January 11, 2013, http://eclkc.ohs.acf.hhs.gov/hslc/tta-system/family/, then clicking on "For Parents," then "Inside Head Start," then "Frequently Asked Questions," and finally "Register for the Program." A recent Google search for "Head Start How Do I Apply" yielded the "Register for the Program" page as the first result.

43. Ibid.
44. "What You Should Know about Head Start," Administration for Children and Families, last reviewed September 2010, accessed January 11, 2013; go to http://eclkc.ohs.acf.hhs.gov/hslc/tta-system/family and click on "For Parents," then "Inside Head Start," then "Frequently Asked Questions," and finally "What You Should Know about Head Start." A recent Google search for "What You Should Know about Head Start" yielded the web page as the first result.
45. "What Is Head Start?" Administration for Children and Families, last reviewed May 2010, accessed January 11, 2013; go to http://eclkc.ohs.acf.hhs.gov/hslc/tta-system/family, and click on "For Parents," then "Inside Head Start," then "Frequently Asked Questions," and finally "What is Head Start?" A recent Google search for "What Is Head Start" yielded the web page as the first result.
46. "What Would Be Your Child's Routine in a Head Start Program?" Administration for Children and Families, last reviewed November 2008, accessed January 11, 2013; go to http://eclkc.ohs.acf.hhs.gov/hslc/tta-system/family, and click on "For Parents," then "Inside Head Start," then "Frequently Asked Questions," and finally "What Would Be Your Child's Routine in a Head Start Program?" A recent Google search for "What Would Be Your Child's Routine in a Head Start Program?" yielded the web page as the first result.
47. *Head Start: Supporting Success for Children and Families* (National Women's Law Center, November 2011), 2, http://www.nwlc.org/sites/default/files/pdfs/head_start_fact_sheet_2011.pdf.
48. W. Steven Barnett et al., *The State of Preschool 2011* (National Institute for Early Education Research, 2011), 5, http://nieer.org/sites/nieer/files/2011yearbook.pdf. This publication also includes data on every state.
49. Ibid., 6.
50. Ibid., 4.
51. "States with Quality Rating and Improvement Systems," National Association for the Education of Young Children, accessed January 11, 2013, http://www.naeyc.org/policy/StateQRIS.
52. Karen Schulman et al., *A Count for Quality: Child Care Center Directors on Rating and Improvement Systems* (National Women's Law Center and CLASP, 2012), 7, http://www.nwlc.org/sites/default/files/pdfs/ACountforQualityQRISReport.pdf.
53. "Flexible Work Arrangements," The Sloan Center on Aging and Work, accessed January 11, 2013, http://workplaceflexibility.bc.edu/types/types_arrangement.
54. "Why Employers Need Workplace Flexibility," The Sloan Center on Aging and Work, accessed January 11, 2013, http://workplaceflexibility.bc.edu/need/need_employers.
55. *Work–Life Balance and the Economics of Workplace Flexibility* (Executive Office of the President: Council of Economic Advisers, March 2010), http://www.whitehouse.gov/files/documents/100331-cea-economics-workplace-flexibility.pdf.
56. "Why Employees Need Workplace Flexibility," The Sloan Center on Aging and Work, accessed January 11, 2013, http://workplaceflexibility.bc.edu/need/need_employees.
57. For citations and even more arguments, please see A Better Balance's fact sheet, *The Business Case for Workplace Flexibility* (A Better Balance, November 2010), http://abetterbal-

ance.org/web/images/stories/Documents/fairness/factsheets/BC-2010-A_Better_Balance.pdf.

58. Ellen Galinsky et al., *Workplace Flexibility: A Guide for Employees* (Families and Work Institute, When Work Works), http://familiesandwork.org/3w/tips/downloads/employees.pdf.
59. "Guide: Flexible Working," Government of the United Kingdom, last updated January 9, 2013, accessed January 14, 2013, https://www.gov.uk/flexible-working/making-a-statutory-application.
60. Anna Danziger and Shelley Waters Boots, *Memo on the Impact of the United Kingdom's Flexible Working Act* (Workplace Flexibility 2010, Memos and Fact Sheets, April 30, 2008), http://scholarship.law.georgetown.edu/legal/12/.
61. Cali Yost, *Work + Life: Finding the Fit That's Right for You* (Riverhead Hardcover, 2004).
62. Ibid., 9.
63. For sample bargaining language, check out the Labor Project for Working Families at http://www.working-families.org/network/bargaining.html.
64. Joan C. Williams, *One Sick Child Away from Being Fired: When "Opting Out" Is Not an Option* (WorkLife Law, University of California Hastings College of Law, 2006), 30, http://www.worklifelaw.org/pubs/onesickchild.pdf.
65. Ellen Galinsky et al., *Workplace Flexibility*.
66. *Workflex Employee Toolkit* (When Work Works, October 2012), http://whenworkworks.org/research/workflexemployeetoolkit.html.
67. Ellen Galinsky et al., *Workplace Flexibility*.
68. Working Families Flexibility Act, S. 2142 112th Cong. (2012), http://www.govtrack.us/congress/bills/112/s2142.
69. Amy Richman et al., *Innovative Workplace Flexibility Options for Hourly Workers* (Corporate Voices for Working Families, May 2009), 4, http://www.cvworkingfamilies.org/system/files/CVWFflexreport-FINAL.pdf.
70. Liz Watson and Jennifer E. Swanberg, *Flexible Workplace Solutions for Low-Wage Hourly Workers: A Framework for a National Conversation* (Workplace Flexibility 2010, May 2011), 5, http://www.uky.edu/Centers/iwin/LWPolicyFinal.pdf.
71. Ibid., 6.
72. Ibid.
73. Ibid., 19.
74. For case studies of employers who made flexibility for hourly workers work, see Richman et al., *Innovative Workplace Flexibility*.
75. Watson and Swanberg, *Flexible Workplace Solutions*, 24.
76. For ideas on how your workplace can accommodate your needs, see Watson and Swanberg, *Flexible Workplace Solutions*, 25–31.
77. Joan Williams, *Reshaping the Work/Family Debate* (Harvard University Press, 2010).
78. Jennifer Ludden, "The End of 9-to-5: When Work Time Is Anytime," National Public Radio, March 16, 2010, http://www.npr.org/templates/story/story. php?storyId=124705801. For more information about state employers and workplace flexibility: Gregory Fetterman et al., *The Legal Framework for States as Employers-of-Choice in Workplace Flexibility: A Case Study of*

Arizona and Michigan (Work–Life Policy Unit, Civil Justice Clinic, Arizona State University Sandra Day O'Connor College of Law, Fall 2009).

79. Cynthia Calvert, *Family Responsibilities Discrimination: Litigation Update 2010* (Center for Worklife Law, March 2010), 2.
80. Shelley J. Correll, Stephen Benard, and In Paik, "Getting a Job: Is There a Motherhood Penalty?" *American Journal of Sociology* 112, no. 5 (March 2007), http://gender.stanford.edu/sites/default/files/motherhoodpenalty.pdf.
81. *Chadwick v. Wellpoint, Inc.*, 561 F.3d 38, 45–46 (1st Cir. 2009).
82. To learn whether your city or county has a caregiver discrimination law, see Stephanie Bornstien and Robert J. Rathmell, *Caregivers as a Protected Class?: The Growth of State and Local Laws Prohibiting Family Responsibilities Discrimination* (Center for WorkLife Law, December 2009), http:// www.worklifelaw.org/pubs/LocalFRDLawsDetail.html.
83. See, generally, Joan C. Williams, *Unbending Gender: Why Work and Family Conflict and What to Do about It* (Oxford University Press, 1999).
84. Dina Bakst, Jared Make, and Nancy Rankin, *Beyond the Breadwinner: Professional Dads Speak Out on Work and Family* (A Better Balance, June 2011), http://abetterbalance.org/web/images/stories/Documents/valuecarework/Reports/ABB_Rep_BeyondBreadwinner.pdf.
85. *Knussman v. Maryland*, 272 F.3d 625 (4th Cir. 2001).
86. *Strate v. Midwest Bankcentre, Inc.*, 398 F.3d 1011 (8th Cir. 2005).
87. *Fact Sheet: The Gender Wage Gap by Occupation* (Institute for Women's Policy Research, April 2012), www.iwpr.org/publications/pubs/the-gender-wage-gap-by-occupation-1/at_download/file.
88. Stephen Benard, In Paik, and Shelley J. Correll, "Cognitive Bias and the Motherhood Penalty," *Hastings Law Journal* 59 (June 2008): 1359.
89. Sarah Jane Gynn and Audry Powers, *The Top 10 Facts about the Wage Gap: Women Are Still Earning Less Than Men Across the Board* (Center for American Progress, April 2012), http://www.americanprogress.org/issues/2012/04/wage_gap_facts.html.
90. Correll, Benard, and Paik, *American Journal of Sociology* 112:1297.
91. Joan C. Williams and Stephanie Bornstein, "The Evolution of 'FRED': Family Responsibilities Discrimination and Developments in the Law of Stereotyping and Implicit Bias," *Hastings Law Journal* 59 (June 2008): 1311, 1327.
92. "Equal Pay/Compensation Discrimination," US Equal Employment Opportunity Commission, accessed January 11, 2013, http://www.eeoc.gov/laws/types/equalcompensation.cfm.
93. *Pay Secrecy and Paycheck Fairness: New Data Shows Pay Transparency Needed* (Institute for Women's Policy Research, November 2010), www.iwpr.org/press-room/press-releases/pay-secrecy-and-paycheck-fairness-new-data-shows-pay-transparency-needed.
94. *Fact Sheet: Combating Punitive Pay Secrecy Policies*, (National Women's Law Center, April 2012), http://www.nwlc.org/sites/default/files/pdfs/paysecrecyfactsheet.pdf.

STATE-BY-STATE GUIDE

Welcome to the state-by-state guide. As we have said throughout this book, even if a federal law might not protect you, do not despair—a state or local law might be able to help instead or in addition. The one thing you should keep in mind is that no matter which state you live in, the federal law applies to almost everyone and is a floor on which states and localities can build if they choose to pass better laws. The purpose of this section is to flag issues for you at the state and local levels. Please note that this is absolutely not an exhaustive list of every single law that might be able to benefit you. This is just a jumping-off point for a discussion with a lawyer who can truly walk you through your rights and entitlements. This caveat is important not only because we might have left off a law that can help you, but also because laws sometimes work out differently in practice from how they are written on paper. You might find out that a law is interpreted differently by a court or state agency, for example. Legal protections are, unfortunately, too complicated for a simple guide like this, so you absolutely must get legal advice tailored to your specific situation by a local expert. For example, we haven't gone into detail about which laws apply to which workers, so a law we describe might not apply to you because you are a particular type of worker (e.g., a teacher) or because you work part-time. That's why it's so important to check up on whether or not you are protected.

Also, you should know that most laws have something called a "statute of limitations," which means that you have to take action within a certain period of time. We did not include the statute of limitations for each law, so be sure to consult with a lawyer about the timing in your specific circumstance. Otherwise you could be out of luck. Generally speaking, it's better to get moving sooner rather than later when it comes to these things.

We also want to disclose that collectively, we are only authorized to practice law in New York and Tennessee. This state-by-state guide should not be interpreted as legal advice or counsel as to other states where we are not licensed to practice. This is why you should consult with a local attorney to understand how local laws will affect you.

As a final warning, we listed state agencies in the "Call for Help" sections, but we want to let you know that sometimes filing with an agency means you cannot file a lawsuit in court. Speak with an attorney about which venue might be your best option before you file anything.

We were inspired to set up this section like a tourist's guide. Icons correspond with the type of law that the state provides, so that you can get an idea of how family-friendly your state is at a glance. Although we know most people don't get to shop for the state they end up living in, we hope that you will be encouraged to advocate in your hometown for better policies. Why should just California have all the fun? Your voice is powerful; if you would like to make sure that families in your state have the same beneficial policies as a neighboring jurisdiction, then contact your legislators. This information is up-to-date as of May 30, 2014. Please check back at our website, www.abetterbalance.org, for updates on this state survey; after all, laws are always changing.

KEY TO THE STATE-BY-STATE GUIDE

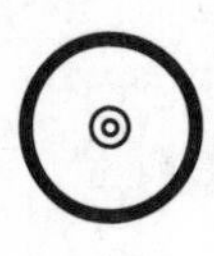

BREASTFEEDING

States have varying types of breastfeeding laws. We have tried to include the laws that we thought would be most helpful to breastfeeding workers, such as laws that require employers to provide break time for pumping or laws that grant women a right to breastfeed in public. We didn't bother including laws that don't count breastfeeding as indecent exposure (talk about the Stone Age!) and other more obscure laws, such as those excusing breastfeeding mothers from jury duty.[1]

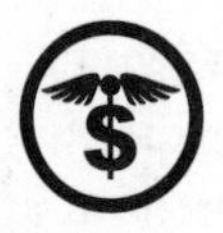

TEMPORARY DISABILITY INSURANCE

Temporary disability insurance (TDI) allows women who are disabled by pregnancy or childbirth to get some wage replacement since they can't work. Only five lucky states have this provision–read on to find out which ones they are.

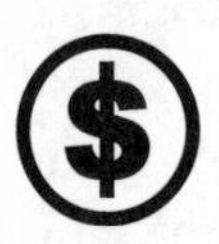

PAID FAMILY LEAVE

Paid family leave (also known as family leave insurance) laws allow workers to use the state's temporary disability insurance fund to receive wage replacement while caring for certain family members, such as a newborn child or ill spouse. Only three states have this.

UNPAID FAMILY LEAVE

Unpaid family leave means that a state goes above and beyond the Family and Medical Leave Act (FMLA) in some way–perhaps workers can take more than twelve weeks off.

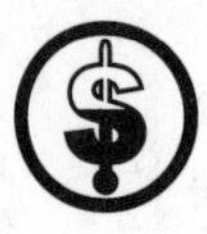

PAID SICK DAYS

Some localities and one state guarantee certain workers time off when they or a family member are sick. This section focuses on those laws.

[1]For comprehensive breastfeeding laws, check out the National Council of State Legislatures: http://www.ncsl.org/issues-research/health/breastfeeding-state-laws.aspx.

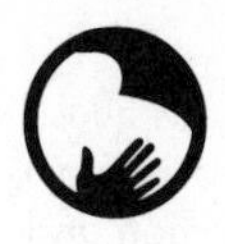

PREGNANCY

In this section we have included laws that help pregnant women–they might let you transfer to a less hazardous position or prohibit pregnancy discrimination. Of course, the federal Pregnancy Discrimination Act (PDA) also protects against pregnancy discrimination, but it can sometimes be helpful to use state and federal laws together–or the state law might apply where the federal doesn't because the employer is so small.

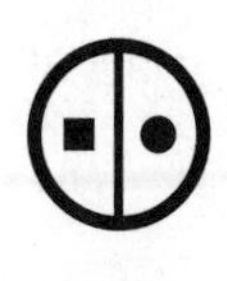

CAREGIVER DISCRIMINATION

Here we have included prominent cities and counties within the state (or occasionally the entire state itself) that protect parents or caregivers from discrimination.[2]

PARENTAL INVOLVEMENT IN CHILDREN'S EDUCATION

Some states let parents take time off to attend school events, such as parent-teacher conferences or other activities. We included those laws and similar ones in this section.

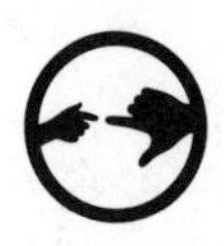

KINCARE

Kincare is a term that means caring for a family member. Kincare laws, which are included in this section, mean that workers are allowed to use their own sick days to care for certain family members.

PUBLIC-SECTOR WORKERS

Unfortunately, we couldn't include every benefit that public-sector workers get in various states, since these laws are extremely complicated and apply differently to different workers. We did try where we could to include examples of helpful additional benefits that public-sector workers have. Check with your employee handbooks, human resources, and union representatives to learn about your rights.[3]

[2]We didn't include every locality; take a look here for updated information: http://www.worklifelaw.org/pubs/LocalFRDLawsDetail.html.

[3]This resource includes many public-sector benefits: http://www.nationalpartnership.org/site/DocServer/Expecting_Better_Report.pdf?docID=10301.

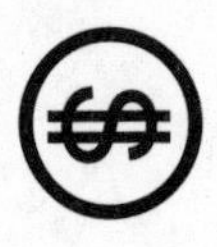

EQUAL PAY

The Equal Pay Act is a federal law, but often states have a statewide equivalent (with sometimes stronger protections) that guarantees equal pay for equal work between men and women. This section includes these state laws.[4]

UNEMPLOYMENT INSURANCE

Unemployment insurance law can be very complicated. The standards for getting unemployment insurance are different from other laws. You might not be able to sue your employer for caregiver discrimination, for example, but you might at least be able to get unemployment if you had to leave work because you couldn't do your caregiving responsibilities and keep your job.[5]

OTHER

This is just for anything else that we thought pregnant women and parents would like to know about. States get bonus points for helping out working families in creative ways.

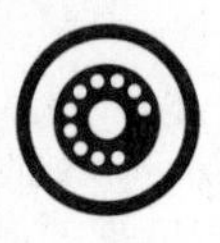

CALL FOR HELP

We included the phone numbers and addresses of state agencies so that you know whom to call to complain about possible violations of the law or to ask questions. Your city or state might also have organizations that can help you.

[4]This resource from the National Conference of State Legislatures features every state's equal pay laws: http://www.ncsl.org/issues-research/labor/equal-pay-laws.aspx.

[5]For more information on how unemployment insurance works for working parents, visit http://nelp.3cdn.net/ebba1e75e059fc749d_0um6idptk.pdf. Page 59 of this report includes more updated information: http://www.nationalpartnership.org/site/DocServer/Expecting_Better_Report.pdf?docID=10301.

ALABAMA

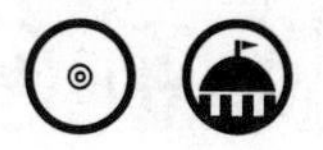

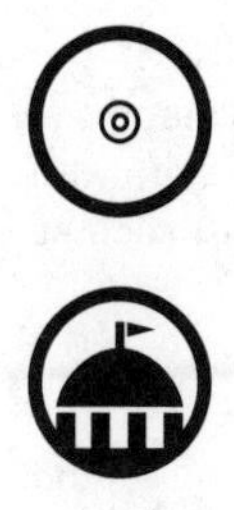

BREASTFEEDING

A mother can breastfeed her child in any location as long as she is allowed to be there.[1]

PUBLIC-SECTOR WORKERS

As a government employee, you may be entitled to more generous benefits, such as the option to use accrued sick time to care for family members.[2] Be sure to check your employee handbook or union contract or talk with human resources.

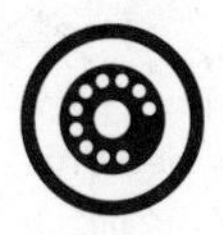

CALL FOR HELP

For questions about breastfeeding laws, you may contact the Alabama Department of Public Health:

Website: http://www.adph.org/contactus.asp?id=498

You may also contact the Alabama Department of Human Resources–Equal Employment and Civil Rights Division:

Phone: 334-242-1550
Website: dhr.alabama.gov/directory/Equal_Emp_Civil_Rts.aspx

[1]Ala. Code § 22-1-13.
[2]Ala. Admin. Code r. 670-X-14-.01.

ALASKA

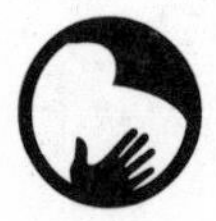

PREGNANCY

Alaska law protects pregnant women from employment discrimination.[1] The law applies to all employers in the state with one or more employees (there are some exceptions, such as for nonprofit religious associations).[2]

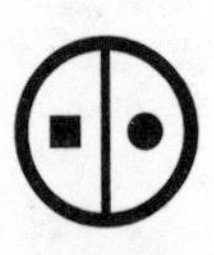

CAREGIVER DISCRIMINATION

Alaska also protects parents from discrimination in the workplace.[3]

PUBLIC-SECTOR WORKERS

As a government employee, you may be entitled to more generous benefits, such as the option to use accrued personal leave to care for an immediate family member's medical disability or for pregnancy/childbirth.[4] You might also be able to transfer to a different position while you are pregnant, if your doctor recommends it.[5] Be sure to check your employee handbook or union contract or talk with human resources.

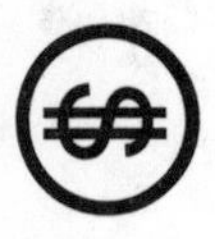

EQUAL PAY

It is unlawful for an employer to discriminate in wages between men and women for jobs of comparable work.[6]

[1]Alaska Stat. § 18.80.220(a).
[2]Alaska Stat. § 18.80.300(5).
[3]Alaska Stat. § 18.80.220(a).
[4]Alaska Stat. § 39.20.225.
[5]Alaska Stat. § 39.20.520.
[6]Alaska Stat. § 18.80.220(a)(5).

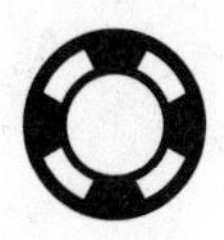

UNEMPLOYMENT INSURANCE

Leaving work to take care of an immediate family member who has a disability or illness may count as "good cause" to quit your job, for the purposes of unemployment benefits.[7]

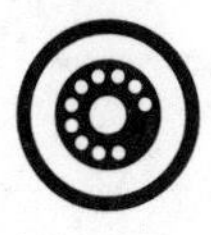

CALL FOR HELP

For questions about the law, or to file a complaint, you may contact the Alaska State Commission for Human Rights:

Phone: 800-478-4692 / TDD 800-478-3177
Address:
Alaska State Commission for Human Rights
800 A Street, Suite 204
Anchorage, AK 99501-3669
Website: humanrights.alaska.gov

[7]Alaska Admin. Code title 8, § 85.095(c)(2).

ARIZONA

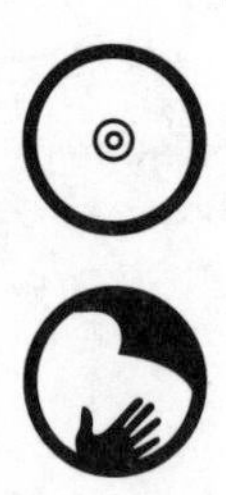

BREASTFEEDING

Mothers may breastfeed in any public or private place wherever they are allowed to be.[1]

PREGNANCY

The Arizona Civil Rights Act protects employees from discrimination on the basis of sex, which probably includes pregnancy.[2] The law applies to employers who have fifteen or more employees.[3]

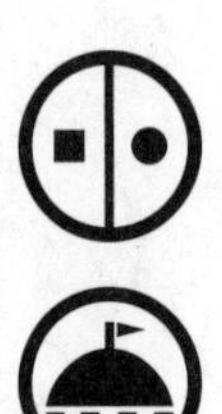

CAREGIVER DISCRIMINATION

In Tucson, employees are protected from discrimination based on family status (parenthood).[4]

PUBLIC-SECTOR WORKERS

As a government employee, you may be entitled to more generous benefits–for example, a parent may opt to take parental leave unpaid and preserve other paid leave days for later use.[5] Be sure to check your employee handbook or union contract or talk with human resources.

[1] Ariz. Rev. Stat. § 41-1443.

[2] Ariz. Rev. Stat. § 41-1463(B). A recent court decision implied that Arizona's definition of "sex" in the law included pregnancy. See Lespron v. Tutor Time Learning Center, LLC, No. CV 10-01760-PHX-NVW, 2012 WL 135978 at *4 (D. Ariz. January 18, 2012) ("Title VII's definition of discrimination based on sex includes pregnancy. The ACRA includes similar prohibitions" [citations omitted]).

[3] Ariz. Rev. Stat. § 41-1461(6).

[4] Tucson, Ariz., Code §§ 10-18(a); 17-11(g).

[5] Ariz. Admin. Code § R2-5-411(B).

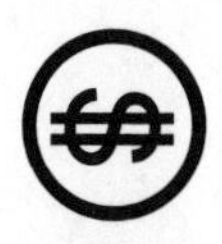

EQUAL PAY

Employers must pay men and women the same wage rates for the same work.[6]

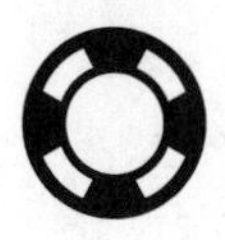

UNEMPLOYMENT INSURANCE

If you had to leave work because of child care issues or to care for an ill family member, you might still be entitled to unemployment benefits[7]–the statute mentions a range of factors to analyze.

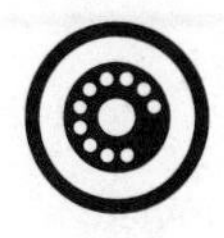

CALL FOR HELP

For questions about the law, or to file a complaint, you may contact the Civil Rights Division of the Arizona Attorney General's Office:

Phone: 602-542-5263 / TDD 602-542-5002
Website: www.attorneygeneral.state.az.us
Email: civilrightsinfo@azag.gov

[6]Ariz. Rev. Stat. § 23-341
[7]Ariz. Rev. Stat. § 23-341.

ARKANSAS

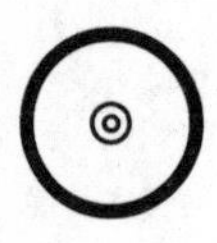

BREASTFEEDING

Arkansas expressly authorizes that women can breastfeed children in public places where other individuals are present.[1]

Your employer has to provide reasonable unpaid break time and make a reasonable effort to provide a location (not a toilet stall) for pumping breast milk.[2]

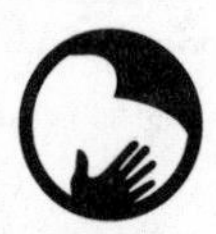

PREGNANCY

The Arkansas Civil Rights Act prohibits sex discrimination[3] inclusive of pregnancy.[4]

PUBLIC-SECTOR WORKERS

As a government employee, you may be entitled to more generous benefits, such as the option to take up to six months off from work using any combination of sick leave, annual leave, and unpaid leave.[5] Be sure to check your employee handbook or union contract or talk with human resources.

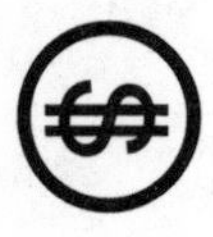

EQUAL PAY

Arkansas has an equal pay law that requires employers to provide equal compensation for equal services.[6]

[1]Ark. Code § 20-27-2001.
[2]Ark. Code § 11-5-116.
[3]Ark. Code § 16-123-107
[4]Ark. Code § 16-123-102
[5]Ark. Code § 21-4-210.
[6]Ark. Code §§ 11-4-601; 11-4-610.

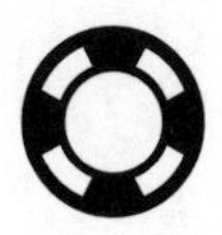

UNEMPLOYMENT INSURANCE

If you left work because of your own or an immediate family member's pregnancy or disability, then you can probably still qualify for unemployment benefits.[7]

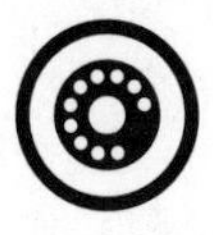

CALL FOR HELP

For wage discrimination questions, you may contact the Arkansas Department of Labor:

Phone: 501-682-4500
Address:
10421 West Markham Street
Little Rock, AR 72205
Email: asklabor@arkansas.gov

[7] Ark. Code § 11-10-513(b)(2).

CALIFORNIA

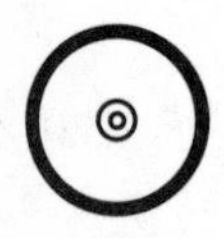

BREASTFEEDING

Moms have a right to breastfeed their children anywhere, public or private (other than someone else's private home), as long as they are authorized to be there in the first place.[1]

Employers have to give you a reasonable amount of break time for expressing breast milk.[2] They also have to try to find a private place for you to pump, other than a toilet stall.[3]

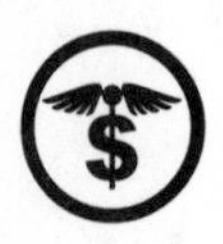

TEMPORARY DISABILITY INSURANCE

California has a temporary disability insurance system, known as State Disability Insurance (SDI), which will provide part of your salary while you are disabled because of pregnancy.[4] Typically, you can get four weeks before your delivery date and up to six weeks afterward for a normal pregnancy.[5]

However, you can get more time with a doctor's certification.

[1]Cal. Civ. Code § 43.3.

[2]Cal. Lab. Code § 1030.

[3]Cal. Lab. Code § 1031.

[4]Cal. Unemp. Ins. Code § 2626. The ways that disability insurance, paid leave, unpaid leave, and the FMLA all interplay can be very complicated and confusing. Be sure to speak with a lawyer about your specific situation and to understand these intertwining laws. Please consult this chart to understand all the different family and pregnancy leave laws: http://www.fehc.ca.gov/act/pdf/California_Leave_Entitlement.pdf.

[5]"FAQ—Pregnancy," State of California Employment Development Department, accessed January 11, 2013, http://www.edd.ca.gov/disability/FAQ_DI_Pregnancy.htm. Find out about your eligibility here: "Disability Insurance Eligibility," State of California Employment Development Department, accessed January 11, 2013, http://www.edd.ca.gov/disability/DI_Eligibility.htm.

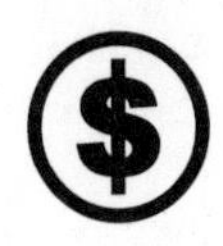

PAID FAMILY LEAVE

California's Family Temporary Disability Insurance law provides eligible employees with partial wage replacement for up to six weeks for caring for a family member.[6]

This benefit can be used to bond with a new child (including foster or adopted children) within the first year or to care for a child, spouse, domestic partner, parent, sibling, grandparent, grandchild, or parent-in-law who is seriously ill.[7]

The benefit amount is approximately 55 percent of your earnings, up to $1,075 per week (as of January 1, 2014).[8]

UNPAID FAMILY LEAVE

The California Family Rights Act provides for twelve weeks of unpaid leave after the birth of a child; after adoption/foster care placement; for the serious health condition of a child, parent (defined broadly, but excluding parents-in-law), spouse, or domestic partner; or for an employee's own serious health condition, excluding pregnancy or childbirth disability.[9]

The California Family Rights Act has the same eligibility requirements as the FMLA (see chapter 2), but is broader than the FMLA because individuals can take unpaid leave to care for a domestic partner.[10]

[6]Cal. Unemp. Ins. Code §§ 3300-3306.
[7]Cal. Unemp. Ins. Code §§ 2708, 3300-3306. See also http://www.edd.ca.gov/disability/PFL_Eligibility.htm. Here is the FAQ section for more information: http://www.paidfamilyleave.org/faqs/#1.
[8]"Paid Family Leave Benefits," accessed January 11, 2013, http://www.edd.ca.gov/disability/PFL_Benefit_Amounts.htm; Disability Insurance (DI) and Paid Family Leave (PFL) Weekly Benefit Amounts in Dollar Increments (State of California Employment Development Department, January 2013), http://www.edd.ca.gov/pdf_pub_ctr/de2589.pdf.
[9]Cal. Gov't Code § 12945.2.
[10]Cal. Fam. Code § 297.5; please view this chart to understand the differences and overlap of the CFRA and FMLA: http://www.fehc.ca.gov/pdf/fmla-cfraregstable-2.pdf.

Eligible workers may take twelve weeks of bonding leave under the California Family Rights Act in addition to four months of pregnancy disability leave. (See below.)

Health insurance must be continued throughout California Family Rights Act leave.[11]

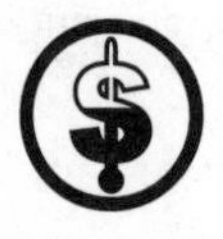

PAID SICK DAYS

The San Francisco Paid Sick Leave Ordinance requires that employees get up to seventy-two hours (nine days) of accrued paid sick time (forty hours for small businesses with fewer than ten employees).[12] Leave can be used for a worker's own or family's medical needs, including routine care.

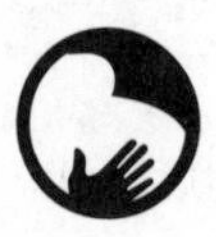

PREGNANCY

For employers with five or more employees:

- Employers in California have to let you take time off (generally up to four months and maybe even more) while you are disabled by pregnancy, childbirth, or a related medical condition; this is often called pregnancy disability leave.[13]
- They have to let you keep your health insurance during this leave.[14]
- Your employer has to accommodate many needs at work that you have because of pregnancy or childbirth, if you ask for the accommodation with the advice of your doctor.[15] (For example, they might have to give you a chair to sit in if your doctor has told you to keep off your feet.)
- You can also get a transfer to a less strenuous or hazardous position because of pregnancy–if the transfer is

[11]Cal. Gov't Code § 12945.2(f).

[12]San Francisco Admin. Code Chap. 12W et seq. Visit here for more information: http://sfgsa.org/index.aspx?page=419.

[13]Cal. Gov't Code § 12945(a)(1).

[14]Cal. Gov't Code § 12945(a)(2).

[15]Cal. Gov't Code § 12945(a)(3)(A).

reasonable (for example, they don't have to create an entirely new position for you).[16]

California law prohibits pregnancy discrimination,[17] and prohibits pregnancy-based harassment by employers with one or more employees.[18]

For more information on all of these provisions, check out the regulations from the California Fair Employment and Housing Commission.[19]

PARENTAL INVOLVEMENT IN CHILDREN'S EDUCATION

If you work for an employer who has twenty-five or more employees, then your boss can't discriminate against you for taking off up to forty hours each year (although no more than eight hours per month) for participating in activities at your child's school or licensed day care.[20] Note that there are a lot of specifics to this law, so look it up and read it carefully.

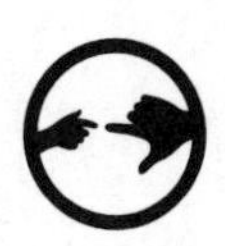

KINCARE

Employees can use up to half of their accrued sick time per year to care for a sick family member (if their employer provides sick leave).[21]

The San Francisco Paid Sick Leave Ordinance lets employees use their accrued time to care for most relatives.[22]

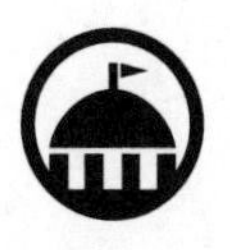

PUBLIC-SECTOR WORKERS

As a government employee, you may be entitled to different benefits. Be sure to check your employee handbook or union contract or talk with human resources.

[16]Cal. Gov't Code §§ 12945(a)(3)(B); 12945(a)(3)(C).
[17]Cal. Gov't Code §§ 12940(a);12926(q).
[18]Cal. Gov't Code § 12940(j).
[19]Cal. Code Regs. title 2, § 7291.
[20]Cal. Lab. Code § 230.8.
[21]Cal. Lab. Code § 233.
[22]San Francisco Admin. Code Chap. 12W.4(a). Visit here for more information: http://sfgsa.org/index.aspx?page=419.

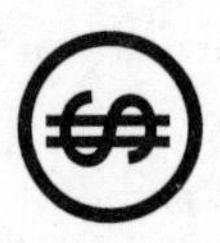

EQUAL PAY

Employees are allowed to tell others how much money they make at work–your boss can't discipline you for doing this.[23]

Employers must pay equal wages for equal work.[24]

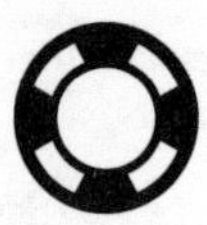

UNEMPLOYMENT INSURANCE

It is considered good cause to leave your work, for unemployment insurance purposes, if you did so because of the health or welfare of your family.[25]

OTHER

San Francisco's new Family Friendly Workplace Ordinance[26] requires that employers with twenty or more employees allow any employee who is employed in San Francisco, has been employed for six months or more by the current employer, and works at least eight hours per week on a regular basis to request a flexible or predictable working arrangement to assist with caregiving responsibilities, including care for:

- a child or children under the age of eighteen;
- a person or persons with a serious health condition in a family relationship with the employee; or
- a parent (age sixty-five or older) of the employee.

An employer who denies a request must explain the denial in a written response that sets out a bona fide business reason for the denial and provides the employee with notice of the right to request reconsideration.

[23]Cal. Lab. Code § 232.
[24]Cal. Lab. Code § 1197.5.
[25]Cal. Code Regs. title 22, § 1256-10.
[26]San Francisco Admin. Code Ch. 127.

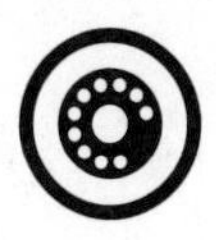

CALL FOR HELP

For questions about disability insurance and paid family leave, contact the State of California Employment Development Department:

Website: http://www.edd.ca.gov/disability/Contact_DI.htm

For discrimination issues, contact the Department of Fair Employment and Housing:

Phone: 800-884-1684 / TDD 800-700-2320
Website: http://www.dfeh.ca.gov
Email: contact.center@dfeh.ca.gov

Other resources:

Equal Rights Advocates
Phone: 415-621-0672
Website: http://www.equalrights.org

The Legal Aid Society Employment Law Center
Phone: 415-864-8848 / TDD 415-593-0091
Website: http://www.las-elc.org

Labor Project for Working Families
Websites:
www.learnworkfamily.org (for union contract language)
www.paidfamilyleave.org (for paid family leave information)

COLORADO

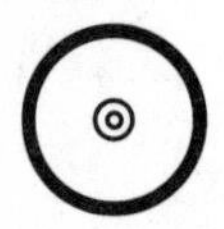

BREASTFEEDING

Colorado permits a woman to breastfeed in any place she has a right to be.[1]

Employers must provide reasonable unpaid break time for expressing breast milk and make a reasonable effort to provide a private space, other than a toilet stall, to pump.[2]

UNPAID FAMILY LEAVE

The Colorado Family Care Act expands the group of family members for whom employees in Colorado may take FMLA leave when the family member has a serious health condition to include a person who is the employee's partner in a civil union or is the employee's domestic partner and either:

- has registered the domestic partnership with the municipality in which the person resides or with the state, if applicable; or
- is recognized by the employer as the employee's domestic partner.

The law will take effect August 7, 2013 (provided it is not subject to referendum petition).[3]

[1]Colo. Rev. Stat. § 25-6-302.
[2]Colo. Rev. Stat. § 8-13.5-104.
[3]Colo. Rev. Stat. § 8-13.3-201-203.

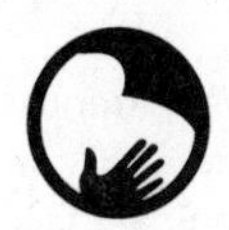

PREGNANCY

The Colorado Anti-Discrimination Act says employers can't discriminate on the basis of sex[4], which includes pregnancy.[5] The Anti-Discrimination Act applies to all employers (even small businesses), including both public and private employers. Religious organizations are not covered by the act unless they accept government funding.[6]

PARENTAL INVOLVEMENT IN CHILDREN'S EDUCATION

For those employers with fifty or more employees, the Parental Involvement in K-12 Education Act lets parents take eighteen hours per year to attend their children's academic activities.[7] Take a look at the law–there are many other provisions to learn about.

PUBLIC-SECTOR WORKERS

As a government employee, you may be entitled to more generous benefits. Be sure to check your employee handbook or union contract or talk with human resources.

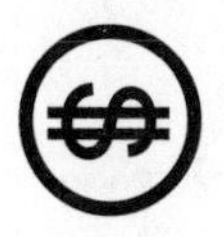

EQUAL PAY

Most employees cannot be disciplined for discussing their wages.[8] Employers also can't discriminate in wages solely on account of sex.[9]

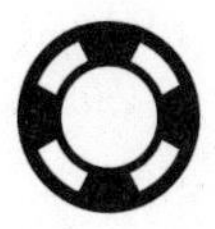

UNEMPLOYMENT INSURANCE

If a worker has to quit because of pregnancy or the health of the employee's spouse or child, then he or she might still qualify for unemployment benefits.[10]

[4]Colo. Rev. Stat. § 24-34-402.
[5]Colorado Civil Rights Com'n v. Travelers Ins. Co., 759 P.2d 1358, 1365 (Colo. 1988). Also take a look at this regulation about pregnancy discrimination: 3 Colo. Code Regs. § 708-1:80.
[6]Colo. Rev. Stat. § 24-34-401(3).
[7]Colo. Rev. Stat. § 8-13.3-101 et seq.
[8]Colo. Rev. Stat. § 24-34-402.
[9]Colo. Rev. Stat. § 8-5-102.
[10]Colo. Rev. Stat. § 8-73-108(4).

OTHER

Colorado law requires employers to treat adoptive parents basically the same as biological parents–for example, if an employer has a policy of providing time off for biological parents after childbirth, then that employer must provide at least that much time off for adoptive parents as well.[11]

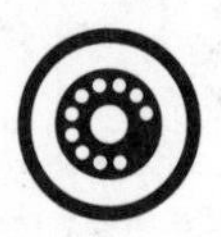

CALL FOR HELP

For questions about the law, or to file a complaint, you may contact the Colorado Civil Rights Division:

Phone: 303-894-2997
Address:
1560 Broadway, Suite 1050
Denver, CO 80202

Other resources:

Colorado Department of Labor and Employment:
Phone: 303-318-8000
Address:
633 17th Street, Suite 201
Denver CO, 80202-3660

9to5 Colorado, National Association of Working Women
Phone: 800-522-0925
Email: 9to5colorado@9to5.org

[11]Colo. Rev. Stat. § 19-5-211(1.5).

CONNECTICUT

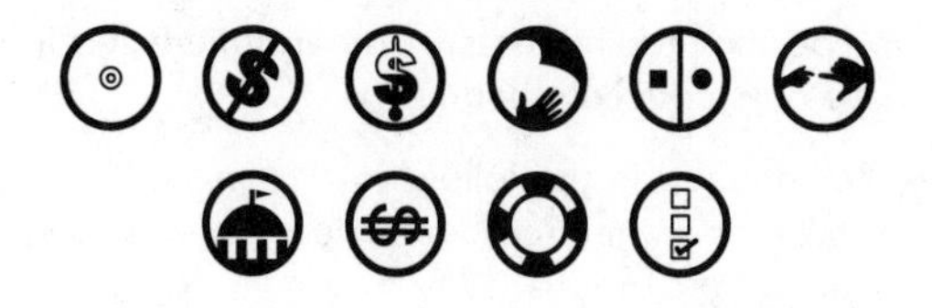

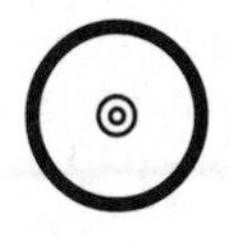

BREASTFEEDING

You are allowed to express breast milk or breastfeed at your work site during your breaks, and your employer can't discriminate against you because you exercise this right.[1]

Employers also have to make reasonable efforts to provide a private area (other than a toilet stall) where breastfeeding women can pump.[2] These laws apply to any employer with one or more employee.[3]

Public places may not restrict a woman's right to breastfeed.[4]

UNPAID FAMILY LEAVE

In addition to FMLA rights for workers in businesses of fifty or more employees, if you work for an employer with seventy-five or more employees, you may be eligible for protection under Connecticut law if you have worked for your employer for twelve months and for a total of one thousand hours in those twelve months (FMLA requires 1250 hours).[5] Eligible employees can also take sixteen weeks of leave during a two-year period[6] (rather than just twelve weeks in a one-year period) for a birth or adoption or to care for a spouse (including same-sex spouses), child, or parent with a serious health condition or for an employee's own serious health condition.[7] Be sure to look

[1]Conn. Gen. Stat. §§ 31-40w(a); 31-40w(c).
[2]Conn. Gen. Stat. § 31-40w(b).
[3]Conn. Gen. Stat. § 31-40w(d).
[4]Conn. Gen. Stat. § 46a-64(a)(3).
[5]Conn. Gen. Stat. § 31-51kk(1), (4).
[6]Conn. Gen. Stat. § 31-51ll(a)(1).
[7]Conn. Gen. Stat. § 31-51ll(a)(2).

up specific requirements if you are interested in intermittent leave or a reduced schedule.

As mentioned in the following "Pregnancy" section, employers have to grant a reasonable leave of absence for disability resulting from pregnancy.[8]

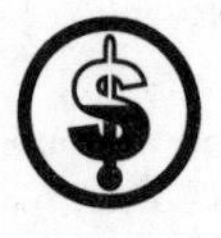

PAID SICK DAYS

Some employers with fifty or more employees are required to provide workers up to forty hours (five days) of accrued sick time per year–which can be used for a spouse or child.[9] Be sure to check carefully to see whether you are covered by this law; a lot of workers are not included.

PREGNANCY

The following laws apply to employers with three or more employees:[10]

- Employers cannot discriminate on the basis of sex,[11] which is specifically defined to include pregnancy, child-bearing capacity, fertility, and other related medical conditions.[12]
- Connecticut law also specifically prohibits employers from firing a woman because of her pregnancy or refusing to grant a reasonable leave of absence when a woman is disabled from pregnancy (she is also entitled to compensation under any disability plan and to return to the same or equivalent job).[13]
- Employers also have to try to transfer pregnant women if the current position puts the fetus at risk (note that the employee has to give written notice of her pregnancy, but the employer also has to let you know about this eligibility requirement).[14]

[8]Conn. Gen. Stat. § 46a-60(a)(7)(b).
[9]Conn. Gen. Stat. § 31-57r et seq.
[10]Conn. Gen. Stat. § 46a-51(10).
[11]Conn. Gen. Stat. § 46a-60(a).
[12]Conn. Gen. Stat. § 46a-51(17).
[13]Conn. Gen. Stat. § 46a-60(a)(7).
[14]Conn. Gen. Stat. § 46a-60(a)(7).

CAREGIVER DISCRIMINATION

As mentioned in the subsequent Other section, employers aren't allowed to ask any job applicant or employee about their family responsibilities, unless it is information directly related to a qualification for the job.[15] However, note that this law does not necessarily protect an employee from discrimination since an employer might find out about responsibilities without asking.

KINCARE

Employees can use up to two weeks of their accumulated sick leave to care for a serious health condition of a child, spouse, or parent or for a birth or adoption if they work for certain employers.[16] This law applies only to employers with seventy-five or more employees.[17]

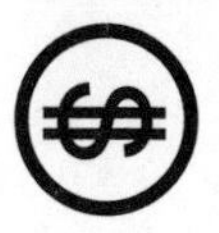

PUBLIC-SECTOR WORKERS

As a government employee, you may be entitled to more generous benefits. Be sure to check your employee handbook or union contract or talk with human resources.

EQUAL PAY

Employers cannot discriminate on the basis of sex in providing compensation.[18]

[15] Conn. Gen. Stat. § 46a-60(a)(9).
[16] Conn. Gen. Stat. § 31-51pp(c)(1).
[17] Conn. Gen. Stat. § 31-51kk(4).
[18] Conn. Gen. Stat. § 31-75.

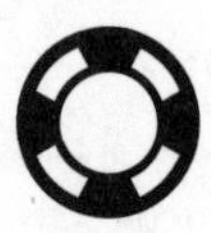

UNEMPLOYMENT INSURANCE

For unemployment insurance purposes, it is considered "good cause" to quit your job if you have to in order to care for your spouse, child, or parent with an illness or disability.[19]

OTHER

Employers aren't allowed to ask any job applicant or employee about their child-bearing age or plans, pregnancy, birth control methods, reproductive system functioning, or family responsibilities, unless it is information directly related to a qualification for the job.[20]

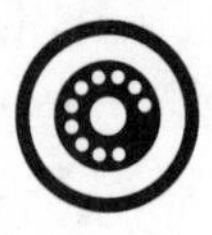

CALL FOR HELP

For questions about state law and to file an employment complaint, you may contact the Commission on Human Rights and Opportunities (CHRO) in Connecticut:

Phone: 800-477-5737 / TDD 860-541-3459
Website: www.ct.gov/chro

[19]Conn. Gen. Stat. § 31-236.

[20]Conn. Gen. Stat. § 46a-60(a)(9). There is an exception in the law for circumstances where workplace exposure to substances might cause birth defects or be hazardous for someone's reproductive system or fetus. Conn. Gen. Stat. § 46a-60(a)(10).

DELAWARE

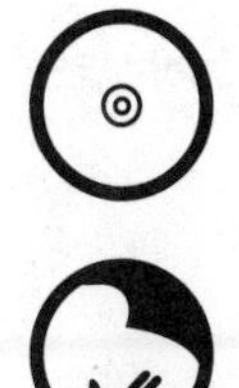

BREASTFEEDING

Delaware permits a mother to breastfeed her child in any location where the mother is permitted to be.[1]

PREGNANCY

The Delaware Discrimination in Employment Act (DDEA) protects from discrimination on the basis of sex.[2] Although the statute does not mention pregnancy, a State of Delaware webpage indicates that pregnancy discrimination is also against the law.[3] The DDEA applies to both private and state organizations with four or more employees.[4]

PUBLIC-SECTOR WORKERS

As a government employee, you may be entitled to different benefits. Be sure to check your employee handbook or union contract or talk with human resources.

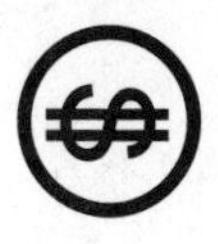

EQUAL PAY

Employees cannot be paid less than coworkers of the opposite sex unless the discrepancy is based on a factor other than sex.[5]

[1]Del. Code title 31, § 310.
[2]Del. Code title 19, § 711(a).
[3]"Pregnancy Discrimination," State of Delaware, last updated October 28, 2012, accessed January 11, 2013, http://dia.delawareworks.com/discrimination/pregnancy.php.
[4]Del. Code title 19, § 710(6).
[5]Del. Code title 19, § 1107A.

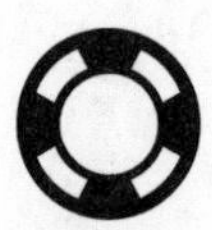

UNEMPLOYMENT INSURANCE

An employee who quits work to care for his or her ill spouse or child can still qualify for unemployment benefits.[6]

CALL FOR HELP

For questions about state law, and to file a complaint, you may contact the Delaware Division of Industrial Affairs:

Phone: 302-761-8200
Address:
4425 North Market Street, 3rd Floor
Wilmington, DE 19802
Website: dia.delawareworks.com/discrimination

[6]Del. Code title 19, § 3314.

DISTRICT OF COLUMBIA

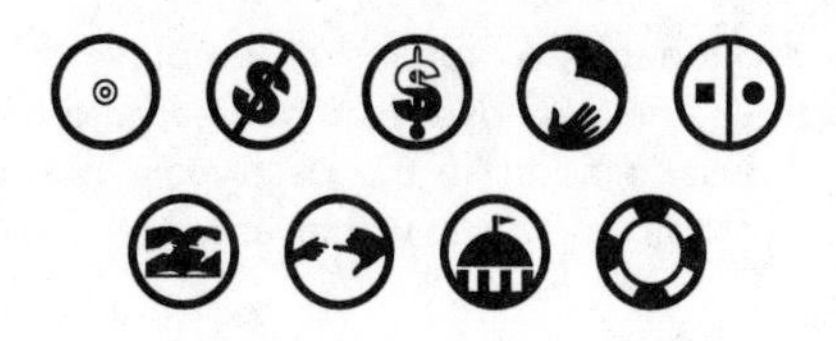

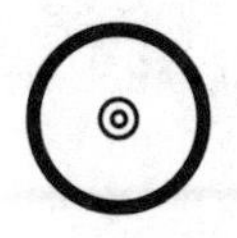

BREASTFEEDING

Women have a right to breastfeed wherever they are otherwise authorized to be.[1]

Employers have to give you reasonable unpaid break periods for pumping breast milk. They also have to try to provide you with a location for pumping other than a toilet stall.[2]

UNPAID FAMILY LEAVE

Employees can get sixteen workweeks of unpaid family leave in a two-year period for a new child or to care for a family member with a serious health issue.[3] The definition of family member under the law is broad, and would include a same-sex spouse or partner.[4] Like the FMLA, this law has many complicated provisions, including details about intermittent leave, reduced schedules, providing your employer with notice, and so on. Take a look at the law and ask for help to make sure you understand everything.

You are entitled to unpaid leave while you are unable to work due to a serious health condition, for up to sixteen weeks in a two-year period.[5]

Employers also have to keep confidential anything about your family relationship that you tell them in order to take advantage of this law.[6]

[1]D.C. Code § 2-1402.82(c).
[2]D.C. Code § 2-1402.82(d).
[3]D.C. Code § 32-502(a).
[4]D.C. Code § 32-501 (4).
[5]D.C. Code § 32-503.
[6]D.C. Code § 32-502(i).

The expanded law applies to employees who have been with the same employer for one year and have accumulated one thousand hours in the past year.[7] It applies to workers employed by employers with twenty or more employees.[8]

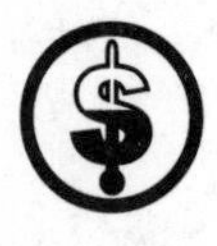

PAID SICK DAYS

Employers with one hundred or more employees have to give each employee accrued sick leave, of up to seven days per year.[9] If the employer has twenty-five to ninety-nine employees, then it has to provide up to five days of accrued sick time.[10] Finally, employers with only twenty-four or fewer employees must give you up to three days of accrued sick leave.[11]

This time can be used for caring for a sick family member.[12]

PREGNANCY

The DC Human Rights Law bans employment discrimination based on sex[13] and clarifies that sex includes pregnancy, childbirth, and breastfeeding.[14] The law also states that pregnant women must be treated the same as other temporarily disabled workers.[15] The law applies to almost all employers.[16]

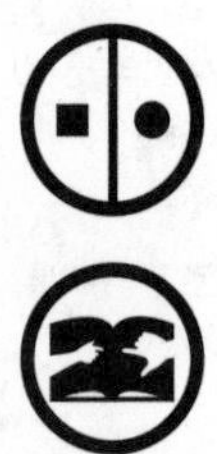

CAREGIVER DISCRIMINATION

DC law prohibits discrimination based on family responsibilities in employment.[17]

PARENTAL INVOLVEMENT IN CHILDREN'S EDUCATION

Under DC law, parents are entitled to twenty-four hours of unpaid leave during a twelve-month period for school-related events for their child.[18] You have to let your employer know you

[7]D.C. Code § 32-501(1).
[8]D.C. Code § 32-516.
[9]D.C. Code § 32-131.02(a)(1).
[10]D.C. Code § 32-131.02(a)(2).
[11]D.C. Code § 32-131.02(a)(3).
[12]D.C. Code § 32-131.02(b)(3).
[13]D.C. Code § 2-1402.11.
[14]D.C. Code § 2-1401.05(a).
[15]D.C. Code § 2-1401.05(b).
[16]D.C. Code § 2-1401.02(10).
[17]D.C. Code § 2-1402.11.
[18]D.C. Code § 32-1202(a).

want time off ten days in advance.[19] "Parent" is defined broadly under the law, (including a grandparent, aunt, or uncle of a child)[20] and "school-related events" includes a lot of different activities.[21]

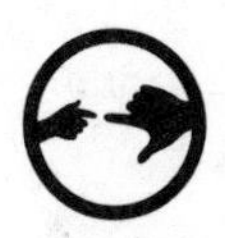

KINCARE

See Paid Sick Days section–employees may use accrued sick leave for family members, but there is not a separate extra kin-care law.

PUBLIC-SECTOR WORKERS

As a government employee, you may be entitled to different benefits. Your rights might depend on whether you work for the federal government or are a different public-sector worker. Be sure to check your employee handbook or union contract or talk with human resources.

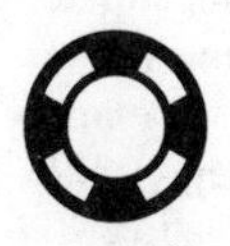

UNEMPLOYMENT INSURANCE

Unemployment benefits can go to someone who leaves their work in order to care for a disabled or ill family member.[22]

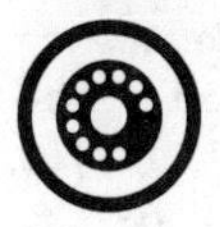

CALL FOR HELP

For questions about the law and to file a claim, you may contact the District of Columbia Office of Human Rights:

Phone: 202-727-4559
Address:
441 4th Street NW, 570 North
Washington, DC 20001
Website: http://ohr.dc.gov
Email: ohr@dc.gov

[19] D.C. Code § 32-1202(e).
[20] D.C. Code § 32-1201(2).
[21] D.C. Code § 32-1201(3).
[22] D.C. Code § 51-110(d)(5).

FLORIDA

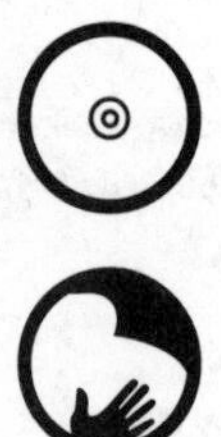

BREASTFEEDING

Florida law allows a mother to breastfeed in any public or private location where she is otherwise allowed to be.[1]

PREGNANCY

The Florida Civil Rights Act prohibits discrimination in employment on the basis of sex.[2] The law applies to employers with fifteen or more employees.[3] The Florida Supreme Court stated in a court ruling that the law does cover pregnancy discrimination. Ask a lawyer to learn more about this.[4]

Some pregnant workers may be protected by Florida laws on disability discrimination. According to the executive director of the Florida Commission on Human Relations, any worker with a "physical or mental impairment that substantially limits one or more major life activities"– meaning that they "cannot perform as well as most people in the general population"– is protected from disability discrimination and may request an accommodation at work. Such an impairment "need not be permanent," so temporary, pregnancy-related conditions "like a 20 pound lifting restriction for several months" may have to be accommodated. Unfortunately, this interpretation is not written into Florida law so ask an attorney for help if you need an accommodation at work.[5]

[1] Fla. Stat. § 383.015.
[2] Fla. Stat. § 760.10.
[3] Fla. Stat. § 760.02(7).
[4] Delva v. The Continental Group, Inc., No. SC12-2315 (Fla., April 17, 2014), available at http://www.floridasupremecourt.org/decisions/2014/sc12-2315.pdf.
[5] Email from Michelle Wilson, executive director of the Florida Commission on Human Relations, to Liz Reiner Platt (Dec. 13, 2013, 17:38 EST) (on file with author).

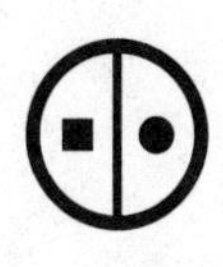

CAREGIVER DISCRIMINATION

A lot of localities in Florida protect caregivers, including Miami-Dade County[6] and Tampa.[7] Check this website to find out whether your city or county provides you with any protections: http://www.worklifelaw.org/pubs/LocalFRDLawsDetail.html.

PUBLIC-SECTOR WORKERS

As a government employee, you may be entitled to more generous benefits, such as six months of unpaid leave for parental or family medical leave.[8] Be sure to check your employee handbook or union contract or talk with human resources.

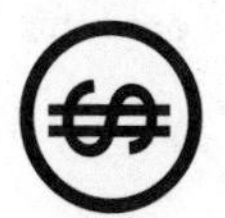

EQUAL PAY

Employers have to pay women the same wages for equal work.[9]

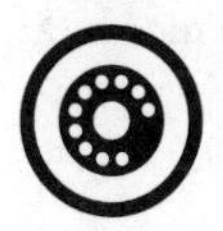

CALL FOR HELP

To find out more about state laws or to file a complaint, you may contact the Florida Commission on Human Relations:

Phone: 850-488-7082 / TDD 800-955-1339
Address:
2009 Apalachee Parkway, Suite 100
Tallahassee, FL 32301
Website: http://fchr.state.fl.us
Email: fchrinfo@fchr.myflorida.com

[6]Miami-Dade County, Fla. Code § 11A-26.
[7]Tampa, Fla. Code § 12-26.
[8]Fla. Stat. § 110.221.
[9]Fla. Stat. § 448.07.

GEORGIA

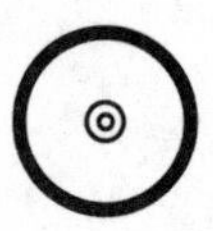

BREASTFEEDING

Mothers are allowed to breastfeed their babies anywhere they are allowed to be.[1]

Georgia law allows employers to provide reasonable unpaid break time in an area other than a toilet stall for employees to pump breast milk–but note that this statute is worded in an odd way; it says employers are allowed to provide this but doesn't seem to require them to.[2] Consult a lawyer about this confusing law.

CAREGIVER DISCRIMINATION

Local Atlanta law protects parents from discrimination at work.[3]

PUBLIC-SECTOR WORKERS

As a government employee, you may be entitled to different benefits. Be sure to check your employee handbook or union contract or talk with human resources.

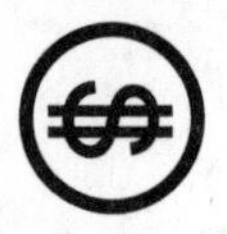

EQUAL PAY

Employers have to pay employees the same rate for equal work.[4]

[1]Ga. Code § 31-1-9.
[2]Ga. Code § 34-1-6.
[3]Atlanta, Ga. Code § 94-112.
[4]Ga. Code § 34-5-3.

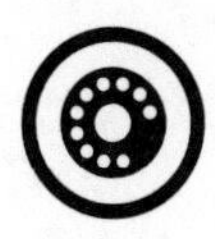

CALL FOR HELP

For questions about state law, you may contact the Georgia Department of Labor:

Phone: 404-232-7300
Website: dol.state.ga.us
Email: dol.state.ga.us/contact_subject.htm

Other resources:

9to5 Atlanta, National Association of Working Women
Phone: 404-222-0037
Address:
501 Pulliam Street SW, Suite 344
Atlanta, GA 30312
Website: 9to5.org

HAWAII

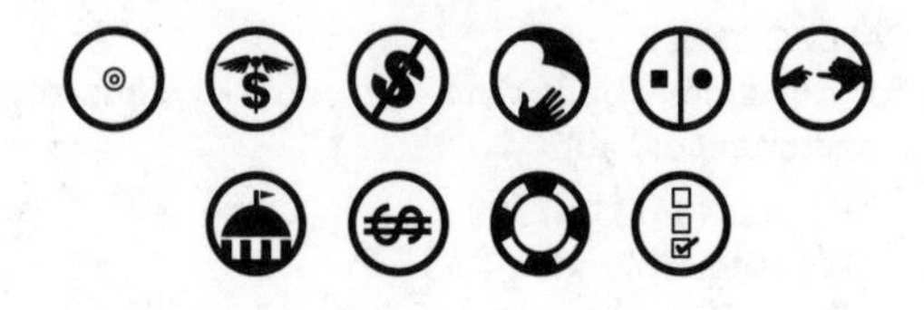

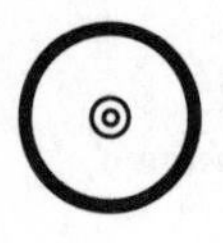

BREASTFEEDING

In Hawaii, it is an act of discrimination for an employer to refuse to hire someone or to fire or penalize an employee because she breastfeeds or expresses breast milk in the workplace.[1]

Also, places of public accommodation cannot discriminate against you because you are breastfeeding.[2]

Employers must provide a reasonable break time for breastfeeding employees to express milk for the employee's nursing child for one year after the child's birth each time the employee has a need to express breast milk. They also must provide a private location that is not a bathroom for employees to express milk. The law contains a hardship exemption for workplaces with fewer than twenty employees, where providing these requirements would be very difficult.[3]

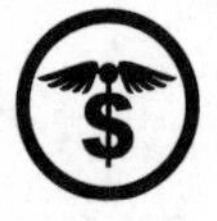

TEMPORARY DISABILITY INSURANCE

Hawaii has a temporary disability insurance program that provides wage-replacement benefits to eligible employees who are disabled because of pregnancy.[4] You can't get the benefits for longer than twenty-six weeks.[5] Be sure to check out the eligibility requirements.[6]

[1]Haw. Rev. Stat. § 378-2(a)(7).
[2]Haw. Rev. Stat. § 489-21.
[3]Haw. Rev. Stat. § 378-92.
[4]Haw. Rev. Stat. § 392-21.
[5]Haw. Rev. Stat. § 392-23.
[6]Haw. Rev. Stat. §§ 392-25; 392-27. Visit this website to learn more about Hawaii's temporary disability insurance laws: http://hawaii.gov/labor/dcd/abouttdi.shtml.

UNPAID FAMILY LEAVE

In addition to FMLA rights for all workers in businesses with fifty or more employees, if you work for an employer with one hundred or more employees and have worked for that employer for at least six months in a row,[7] you are entitled to four weeks of family leave during a calendar year regardless of the number of hours you work for your employer. That leave is available for the birth or adoption of a child or to care for your child, spouse, or parent with a serious health condition or to care for a designated "reciprocal beneficiary," which may include a same-sex partner.[8]

Like the FMLA, this law has many provisions, so take a careful look.

PREGNANCY

It is illegal to discriminate on the basis of sex in employment.[9] Sex is defined to include pregnancy, and the law states that pregnant women have to be treated the same as other similarly situated individuals.[10] It applies to all employers with one or more employees.[11]

There are also regulations stating that you can take off a reasonable period of time (as defined by your doctor) for disability due to pregnancy and childbirth.[12] The regulations also say that the employer must make reasonable accommodations for women affected by disability because of pregnancy or childbirth.[13] According to the deputy executive director of

[7]Haw. Rev. Stat. § 398-1.
[8]Haw. Rev. Stat. § 398-3.
[9]Haw. Rev. Stat. § 378-2(a)(1).
[10]Haw. Rev. Stat. § 378-1.
[11]Haw. Rev. Stat. § 378-1.
[12]Haw. Code R. § 12-46-108.
[13]Haw. Code R. § 12-46-107. Normally we would be hesitant about giving you a regulation instead of the statute itself, but we feel better about these because the Hawaii Supreme Court specifically upheld the right to reasonable leave. See Sam Teague, Ltd. v. Hawai'i Civil Rights Com'n, 971 P.2d 1104 (Hawai'i 1999); see also Noreen Farreell et al., Expecting a Baby, Not a Lay-Off (Equal Rights Advocates, 2012), 29, http://www.equalrights.org/ media /2012/ERA-PregAccomReport.pdf.

the Hawaii Civil Rights Commission, even workers with healthy pregnancies must be allowed preventative accommodation to keep them healthy on the job.[14] Employees may need to provide a doctor's note stating their work restrictions.

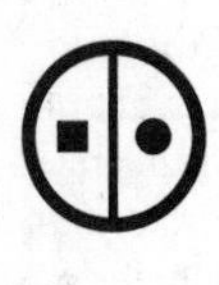

CAREGIVER DISCRIMINATION

In Hawaii, it is illegal for any employer, labor organization, or employment agency to exclude or otherwise deny equal jobs or benefits to a qualified individual because of the known disability of an individual with whom the qualified individual is known to have a relationship or association.[15]

KINCARE

If your employer provides you with sick leave, then you can use that sick time to care for your family, but only up to ten days.[16]

(Take a look at this state's Unpaid Family Leave section–this law is a part of that broader statute.)

PUBLIC-SECTOR WORKERS

As a government employee, you may be entitled to different benefits. Be sure to check your employee handbook or union contract or talk with human resources.

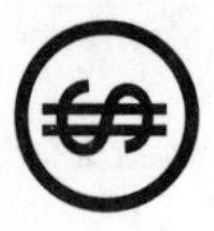

EQUAL PAY

Employers cannot discriminate on the basis of sex in paying wages.[17]

The Hawaii Domestic Workers Bill of Rights prohibits an employer from discriminating against any individual employed

[14]Email from Marcus Kawatachi, deputy executive director of the Hawaii Civil Rights Commission, to Liz Reiner Platt (Feb. 14, 2014 17:01 EST) (on file with author).

[15]Haw. Rev. Stat. § 378-2(a)(6)

[16]Haw. Rev. Stat. § 398-4(c).

[17]Haw. Rev. Stat. § 378-2.3.

as a domestic, in compensation or in terms, conditions, or privileges or employment because of the individual's race, sex (including gender identity or expression), sexual orientation, age, religion, color, ancestry, disability or marital status.[18]

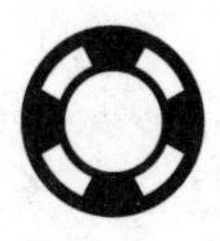

UNEMPLOYMENT INSURANCE

You can't be disqualified from unemployment benefits if you quit for a compelling family reason, meaning an illness or disability of someone in your immediate family, among other things.[19]

OTHER

It is against Hawaii law for your employer to discriminate against you because you are associated with someone who has a disability (such as your child).[20]

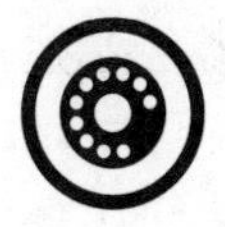

CALL FOR HELP

For more information about the law or to file a complaint, you may contact the Hawaii Civil Rights Commission:

Phone: 808-586-8638/ TDD 808-586-8692
Address:
830 Punchbowl Street, Room 411
Honolulu, HI 96813
Website: hawaii.gov/labor/hcrc
Email: DLIR.HCRC.INFOR@hawaii.gov

[18]Haw. Rev. Stat. § 378-2(a)(9).
[19]Haw. Rev. Stat. § 383-7.6.
[20]Haw. Rev. Stat. § 378-2(a)(6).

IDAHO

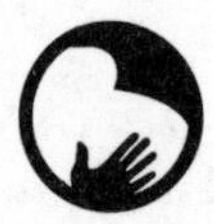

PREGNANCY

Idaho law prohibits sex discrimination in employment.[1] The law applies to employers who have five or more employees.[2] The law might protect against pregnancy discrimination; ask an attorney for help.[3]

PUBLIC-SECTOR WORKERS

As a government employee, you may be entitled to different benefits. Be sure to check your employee handbook or union contract or talk with human resources.

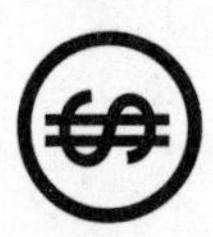

EQUAL PAY

Men and women have to be paid the same for comparable work.[4]

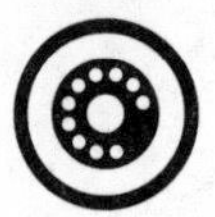

CALL FOR HELP

For more information, and to file a charge, you may contact the Idaho Commission on Human Rights:

Phone: 208-334-2873
Address:
Idaho Commission on Human Rights
317 West Main Street
Boise, ID 83735-0660
Website: humanrights.idaho.gov
Email: inquiry@ihrc.idaho.gov

[1] Idaho Code § 67-5909.
[2] Idaho Code § 67-5902(6).
[3] One woman was successful in winning a lawsuit based on pregnancy discrimination under the Idaho Human Rights Act. See Stout v. Key Training Corp., 158 P.3d 971 (Idaho 2007).
[4] Idaho Code § 44-1702.

ILLINOIS

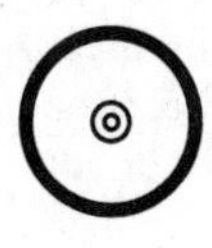

BREASTFEEDING

The Illinois Right to Breastfeed Act provides that a mother may breastfeed wherever she has a right to be, although the law also mentions that a mother should follow the norms of a particular place of worship if she wants to breastfeed there.[1]

Employers with more than five employees must give women breaks to pump breast milk[2] and must try to find employees a private space, other than a toilet stall, to pump.[3]

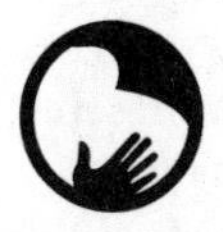

PREGNANCY

The law applies to most employers who have fifteen or more employees.[4]

It is illegal for an employer to discriminate against pregnant women. Women affected by pregnancy or childbirth must be treated the same as other similarly situated workers.[5]

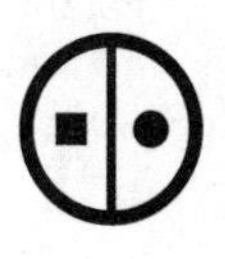

CAREGIVER DISCRIMINATION

There are a few localities that provide protection against caregiver discrimination. For example, in Chicago, parents are protected.[6] For the complete list, visit http://www.worklifelaw.org/pubs/LocalFRDLawsDetail.html.[7]

[1]740 Ill. Comp. Stat. 137/10.
[2]820 Ill. Comp. Stat. 260/10.
[3]820 Ill. Comp. Stat. 260/15.
[4]775 Ill. Comp. Stat. 5/2-101(B)(1)(a).
[5]775 Ill. Comp. Stat. 5/2-102(I).
[6]Chicago, Ill. Code § 2-160-030.
[7]The Illinois Human Rights Commission has also interpreted state law to prohibit (as sex discrimination) employer policies that restrict opportunities for women with minor children. Ill. Admin. Code tit. 56 § 5210.80.

PARENTAL INVOLVEMENT IN CHILDREN'S EDUCATION

The School Visitation Rights Act applies to employers who have at least fifty employees in Illinois.[8]

To be eligible under the School Visitation Rights Act, you must have worked for at least six consecutive months before making a request. You also need to have worked at least half the number of hours that a full-time employee works for your employer.[9]

Eligible employees must be granted up to eight hours of unpaid leave from work per year (although not more than four hours in any given day) in order to attend school conferences or classroom activities for the employee's child, if the activities can't be scheduled during non-work hours. Before you can use this leave time, however, you have to exhaust any vacation, personal, or other compensatory leave (but not sick/disability leave). You have to put a request for leave in writing seven days in advance, or twenty-four hours in advance in the case of emergency.[10]

PUBLIC-SECTOR WORKERS

As a government employee, you may be entitled to different benefits; for example, peace officers and firefighters who are pregnant can be temporarily transferred to a less strenuous or hazardous position.[11]

Be sure to check your employee handbook or union contract or talk with human resources.

[8] 820 Ill. Comp. Stat. 147/40.
[9] 820 Ill. Comp. Stat. 147/10(a).
[10] 820 Ill. Comp. Stat. 147/15.
[11] 775 Ill. Comp. Stat. 5/2-102(H).

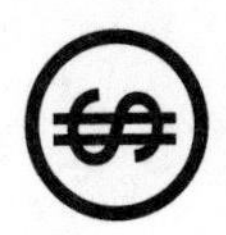

EQUAL PAY

Employers can't pay men and women differently for doing the same or substantially similar work, unless the pay is based on a factor other than sex.[12]

Employers also can't discriminate against you for comparing or discussing your wages.[13]

These laws apply to employers with four or more employees.[14]

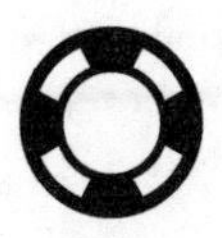

UNEMPLOYMENT INSURANCE

You might still be eligible for unemployment insurance benefits even if you left your work voluntarily if you did so to care for a spouse, child, or parent who is in poor health or disabled.[15]

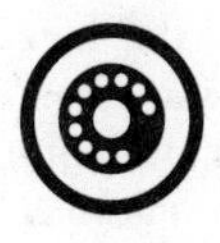

CALL FOR HELP

For more information or to file a complaint of discrimination, you may contact the State of Illinois Human Rights Commission:

Phone: 312-814-6269 / TDD: 312-814-4760
Address:
James R. Thompson Center
100 W. Randolph Street, Suite 5-100
Chicago, IL 60601
Website: www2.illinois.gov/ihrc

[12] 820 Ill. Comp. Stat. 112/10(a).
[13] 820 Ill. Comp. Stat. 112/10(b).
[14] 820 Ill. Comp. Stat. 112/5.
[15] 820 Ill. Comp. Stat. 405/601(B)(1).

INDIANA

BREASTFEEDING

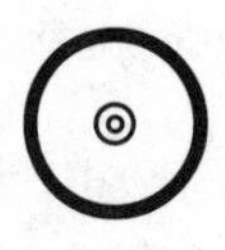

A woman can breastfeed her child anywhere that she has a right to be.[1]

Employers with twenty-five or more employees also have to provide a private space where you can pump breast milk, other than a toilet stall, and provide a refrigerator (or let you bring in a cooler) for the milk, to the extent reasonably possible.[2]

PREGNANCY

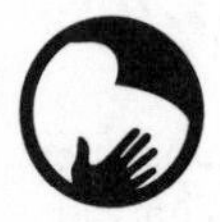

Indiana bans sex discrimination[3] in employment for any employers with six or more employees (although some religious organizations are excluded).[4] Sex discrimination might include pregnancy discrimination; speak with an attorney about this.

PUBLIC-SECTOR WORKERS

As a government employee, you may be entitled to different benefits. Be sure to check your employee handbook or union contract or talk with human resources.

EQUAL PAY

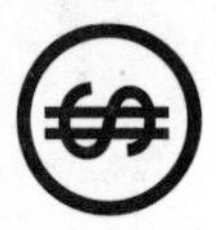

Employers must pay the same wages for equal work in the same establishment.[5]

[1]Ind. Code § 16-35-6-1.
[2]Ind. Code § 22-2-14-2.
[3]Ind. Code § 22-9-1-2.
[4]Ind. Code § 22-9-1-3(h).
[5]Ind. Code § 22-2-2-4(d).

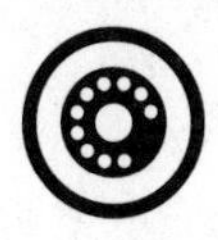

CALL FOR HELP

To learn more about the law or to file a complaint, you may contact the Indiana Civil Rights Commission:

Phone: 317-232-2600 / TDD 800-743-3333
Address:
Indiana Government Center North
100 North Senate Avenue, Room N103
Indianapolis, IN 46204
Website: www.in.gov/icrc

IOWA

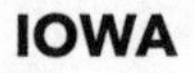

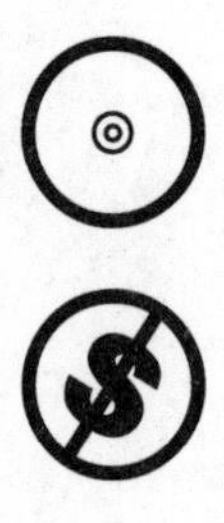

BREASTFEEDING

A woman may breastfeed her child in any public place where she has a right to be.[1]

UNPAID FAMILY LEAVE

In addition to FMLA leave for employers with fifty or more workers, all employers with four or more workers must give their pregnant employees eight weeks to address issues of pregnancy, childbirth, and related disabilities. That leave must be given regardless of job tenure or hours worked.[2]

Note that you have to provide timely notice and might have to certify with a doctor's note that you aren't able to do your job.

PREGNANCY

The Iowa Civil Rights Act prohibits discrimination on the basis of sex,[3] pregnancy, childbirth, and related medical conditions.[4] The law applies to employers with four or more employees.[5]

The law also specifies that disabilities related to pregnancy or childbirth are, for job-related purposes, temporary disabilities and have to be treated the same as any other temporary disabilities.[6]

Even if you are not disabled, you may be entitled to a reasonable accommodation at work under Iowa law. An order of the Iowa Civil Right Commission, Latham v. ABCM Corp., held that

[1]Iowa Code § 135.30A.
[2]Iowa Code § 216.6(2)(e).
[3]Iowa Code § 216.6(1).
[4]See Deboom v. Raining Rose, Inc., 772 N.W. 2d 1, 8 (Iowa 2009), citing Iowa Code § 216.6(2)(d).
[5]Iowa Code § 216.6(6)(a).
[6]Iowa Code § 216.6(2)(b).

"there is a duty to make reasonable accommodations in pregnancy cases."[7] A fact sheet by the Iowa Civil Rights Commission also indicates that this means that pregnant women are entitled to reasonable accommodations at work.[8]

There is no accommodations requirement explicit in Iowa law, however. You should discuss this with a lawyer if you are thinking of bringing a legal challenge against your employer for refusing to accommodate you during pregnancy.

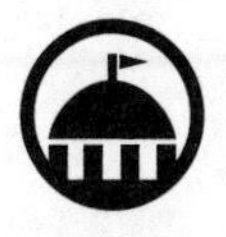

PUBLIC-SECTOR WORKERS

As a government employee, you may be entitled to different benefits. Be sure to check your employee handbook or union contract or talk with human resources.

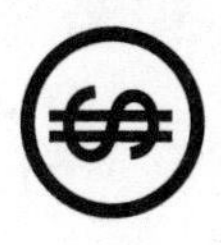

EQUAL PAY

Employers with four or more employees cannot pay men and women in the same establishment different wages for equal work on jobs that are performed under similar working conditions and that require equal skill, effort, and responsibility, unless differential payment is made pursuant to a seniority system, merit system, system which measures earnings by quantity or quality of production, or is based on a factor other than sex.[9]

[7]Order of the Iowa Civil Rights Commission, Latham v. ABCM Corporation, CP# 12-10-60032, DIA No. 12ICRC002, January 24, 2013; Email from Beth Townsend, director of the Iowa Civil Rights Commission, to Liz Reiner Platt (Jan. 21, 2014 15:53 EST) (on file with author).

[8]Pregnancy Factsheet (Iowa Civil Rights Commission, April 2006), http://www.state.ia.us/government/crc/docs/Pregnancy_Factsheet_July08.pdf.

[9]Iowa Code § 216.6A.

UNEMPLOYMENT INSURANCE

You are not disqualified from unemployment benefits if you left work in order to take care of a member of your immediate family who was ill or injured or for pregnancy, although there are other requirements as well.[10]

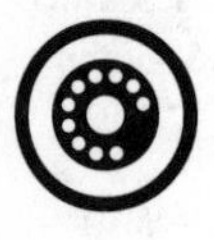

CALL FOR HELP

For questions about the law or to file a complaint, you may contact the Iowa Civil Rights Commission:

Phone: 515-281-4121
Address:
Iowa Civil Rights Commission
Grimes State Office Building
400 E. 14th Street
Des Moines, IA 50319-1004
Website: www.state.ia.us/government/crc

[10]Iowa Code §§ 96.5(1)(c); 96.5(1)(d).

KANSAS

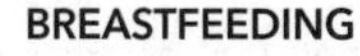

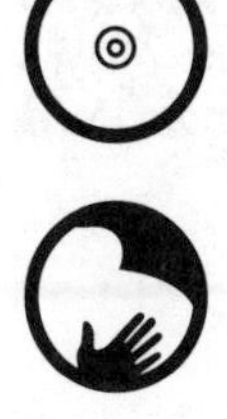

BREASTFEEDING

A mother may breastfeed any place she has a right to be.[1]

PREGNANCY

Kansas prohibits sex discrimination in the workplace.[2]

This law applies to employers with four or more employees.[3]

Pregnancy might be included under sex discrimination; ask a lawyer for help.

An administrative regulation states that childbearing "must be considered by the employer to be a justification for a leave of absence for female employees for a reasonable period of time." An employee who returns to work within a "reasonable" time must be reinstated "to her original job or to a position of like status and without loss of service credits, seniority or other benefits" after childbirth.[4] Furthermore, the Kansas Human Rights Commission's newsletter, Spectrum, noted that employers "may not require that maternity leaves begin or end at predetermined times, without regard to individual capabilities and demands of the particular job."[5]

The Spectrum Newsletter, cited above, also states that under the Kansas Act Against Discrimination, workers with pregnancy-

[1]Kan. Stat. § 65-1,248.
[2]Kan. Stat. § 44-1009.
[3]Kan. Stat. § 44-1002(b).
[4]K.A.R. 21-32-6 (d).
[5]Kansas Human Rights Commission, Spotlight on. . . Pregnancy Discrimination, Spectrum Newsletter (Fall 2011) 3, http://www.khrc.net/SpotlightWeb/Pregnancy_Discrimination.pdf.

related disabilities are entitled to reasonable accommodations at work.[6] Such accommodations could include a temporary leave of absence for workers on bed rest.

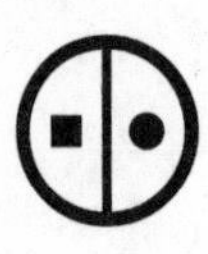

CAREGIVER DISCRIMINATION

There are a few different localities that provide protections for caregivers, such as Leavenworth.[7] Check out http://www.worklifelaw.org/pubs/LocalFRDLawsDetail.html for more information.

PUBLIC-SECTOR WORKERS

As a government employee, you may be entitled to different benefits. Be sure to check your employee handbook or union contract or talk with human resources.

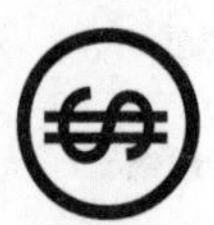

EQUAL PAY

Employers cannot pay men and women in the same establishment different wages for equal work.[8]

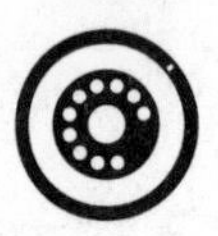

CALL FOR HELP

For questions about the law or to file a complaint, you may contact the Kansas Human Rights Commission:

Phone: 785-296-3206
Address:
900 SW Jackson, Suite 568-S
Topeka, KS 66612-1258
Website: www.khrc.net
Email: khrc@ink.org

[6] Spotlight on . . . Pregnancy Discrimination, Spectrum Newsletter (Fall 2011) at 2.

[7] Leavenworth, Kan. Code § 58-68.

[8] Kan. Stat. § 44-1205.

KENTUCKY

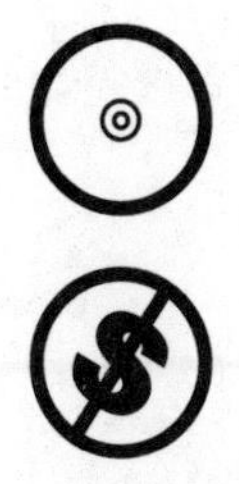

BREASTFEEDING
Moms may breastfeed or pump breast milk in any location where they are allowed to be.[1]

UNPAID FAMILY LEAVE
All employees, regardless of the size of the employer, are entitled to a reasonable leave of absence not to exceed six weeks to care for a recently adopted child under the age of seven.[2]

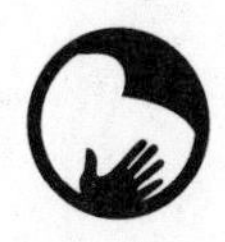

PREGNANCY
Sex discrimination, including pregnancy,[3] is prohibited under Kentucky law.[4] The law applies to all employers with eight or more employees.

PUBLIC-SECTOR WORKERS
As a government employee, you may be entitled to different benefits. Be sure to check your employee handbook or union contract or talk with human resources.

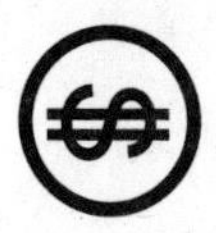

EQUAL PAY
Employees must be paid the same for comparable work in the same establishment.[5]

[1] Ky. Rev. Stat. § 211.755.
[2] Ky. Rev. Stat. § 337.015.
[3] Ky. Rev. Stat. § 344.030(8).
[4] Ky. Rev. Stat. § 344.040.
[5] Ky. Rev. Stat. § 337.423.

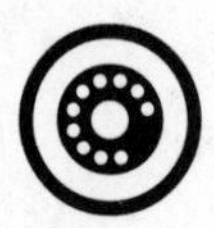

CALL FOR HELP

For questions about the law or to file a complaint, you may contact the Kentucky Commission on Human Rights:

Phone: 502-595-4024 / TDD: 502-595-4084
Address:
332 W. Broadway, 7th Floor
Louisville, KY 40202
Website: kchr.ky.gov
Email: kchr.mail@ky.gov

LOUISIANA

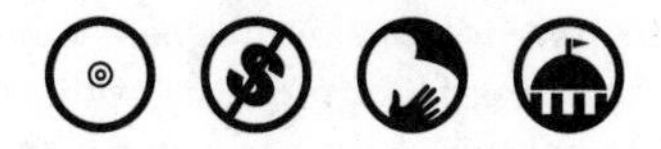

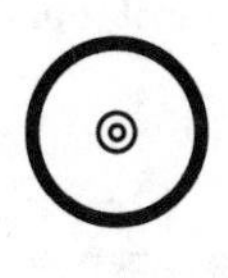

BREASTFEEDING

A mother may breastfeed her baby in any public place.[1]

It is also unlawful for a place of public accommodation (basically, any public place) to discriminate against breastfeeding mothers.[2]

Child care facilities may not discriminate against breastfed babies [3]

UNPAID FAMILY LEAVE

In addition to those covered by FMLA leave, women working for employers with twenty-five or more employees can take up to four months of leave while they are disabled because of pregnancy or childbirth.[4] The law states that employers are not required to give employees disability leave on account of a normal pregnancy/childbirth for more than six weeks.[5]

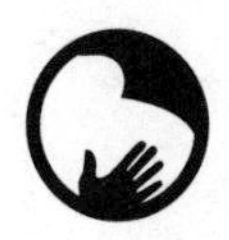

PREGNANCY

Louisiana law specifically protects pregnant women from discrimination in the workplace.[6] This law applies only to employers with more than twenty-five employees.[7]

Louisiana also explicitly states that employers have to treat pregnant women the same as temporarily disabled employees in terms of taking sick leave or other accrued leave.[8]

[1]La. Rev. Stat. § 51:2247.1(B).
[2]La. Rev. Stat. §§ 51:2247.1(C)-(D).
[3]La. Rev. Stat. § 46:1407(B)(1)(e).
[4]La. Rev. Stat. § 23:342(2)(b).
[5]La. Rev. Stat. § 23:341(B)(1).
[6]La. Rev. Stat. § 23:342(1).
[7]La. Rev. Stat. § 23:341(A).
[8]La. Rev. Stat. § 23:342(2)(a).

Employers have to transfer pregnant women to less strenuous or hazardous jobs if they request it with the advice of their physicians (but only when the move can be reasonably accommodated).[9] If the employer already transfers temporarily disabled employees, then it has to let pregnant employees transfer as well.[10]

PUBLIC-SECTOR WORKERS

As a government employee, you may be entitled to different benefits. Be sure to check your employee handbook or union contract or talk with human resources.

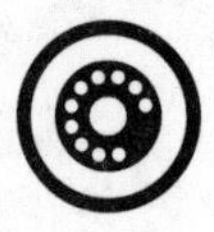

CALL FOR HELP

For questions about the law or to file a complaint, you may contact the Louisiana Commission on Human Rights:

Phone: 225-342-6969 / TDD 1-888-248-0859
Address:
Governor's Office Louisiana Commission of Human Rights
1001 N. 23rd Street, Suite 268
Baton Rouge, LA 70802
Website: gov.louisiana.gov/HumanRights

[9]La. Rev. Stat. § 23:342(4).
[10]La. Rev. Stat. § 23:342(3).

MAINE

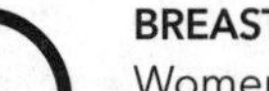

BREASTFEEDING

Women may breastfeed their babies anywhere they have a right to be.[1]

Employers must provide break time for mothers to express breast milk for up to three years following childbirth. The employer has to make reasonable efforts to find you a private place other than the bathroom for pumping and cannot discriminate against you for expressing breast milk in the workplace.[2]

UNPAID FAMILY LEAVE

In addition to those covered by the FMLA, if you work for an employer with fifteen or more employees[3] and have been employed at the same place for one year, then you are entitled to ten weeks of family and medical leave in a two-year period regardless of the number of hours you work.[4] The Maine state law also includes siblings and domestic partners as family members and covers same-sex spouses.[5] Like the FMLA, this law has many provisions, so be sure to take a look if you are interested in taking advantage of your rights.

[1]Me. Rev. Stat. title 5, § 4634.
[2]Me. Rev. Stat. title 26, § 604.
[3]Ibid.
[4]Me. Rev. Stat. title 26, § 844(1).
[5]Me. Rev. Stat. title 26, § 843(4).

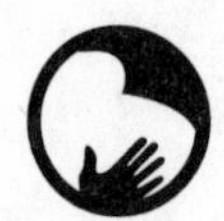

PREGNANCY

Employers may not discriminate against employees on the basis of sex.[6]

Sex includes pregnancy,[7] and the law is clear that pregnant women who are able to work in a different manner must be treated the same as others who can work, and those who cannot work must also be treated the same as other similarly situated employees.[8] According to the commission counsel for the Maine Human Rights Commission, what matters is not how the employer has treated someone who has the exact same limitations as you, but rather "the employer's approach to such conditions generally" such as, for example, whether they have "generally permitted accommodations for other impaired workers."[9] If so, they have to accommodate pregnant workers equally. The law applies to almost all employers.[10]

KINCARE

You can use sick time, vacation time, and comp time that your employer gives you to take care of an ill immediate family member.[11] The law applies to employers with twenty-five or more employees.[12]

PUBLIC-SECTOR WORKERS

As a government employee, you may be entitled to different benefits. Be sure to check your employee handbook or union contract or talk with human resources.

[6] Me. Rev. Stat. title 5, § 4572.
[7] Me. Rev. Stat. title 5, § 4572-A(1).
[8] Me. Rev. Stat. title 5, §§ 4572-A(2); 4572-A(3).
[9] Email from Barbara Archer Hirsch, commission counsel of the Maine Human Rights Commission, to Liz Reiner Platt (Jan. 10, 2014 15:19 EST) (on file with author).
[10] Me. Rev. Stat. title 5, § 4553(4).
[11] Me. Rev. Stat. title 26, §§ 636(1); 636(2).
[12] Me. Rev. Stat. title 26, § 636(1)(A).

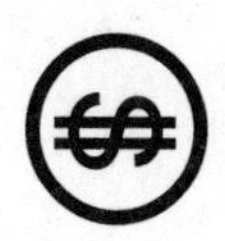

EQUAL PAY

Employers cannot discriminate on the basis of sex in the same establishment for comparable work.[13]

Also, an employer can't stop you from disclosing your wages or asking a coworker about their wages if you are discussing wages in order to enforce your right to equal pay.[14]

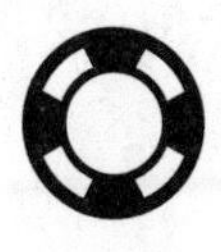

UNEMPLOYMENT INSURANCE

If you left work because of an illness or disability in your immediate family, and your employer couldn't (or wouldn't) accommodate you, then you might still be eligible for benefits.[15]

OTHER

Maine protects employees from discrimination because of a relationship or association with someone who has a disability.[16]

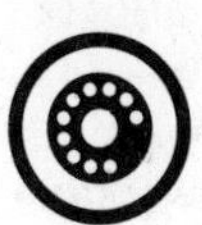

CALL FOR HELP

For questions about the law or to file a complaint, you may contact the Maine Human Rights Commission:

Phone: 207-624-6290 / TTY: Maine Relay 711
Address:
51 State House Station
Augusta, ME 04333
Website: www.maine.gov/mhrc

[13]Me. Rev. Stat. title 26, § 628.
[14]Me. Rev. Stat. title 26, § 628.
[15]Me. Rev. Stat. title 26, § 1193(1)(A)(1).
[16]Me. Rev. Stat. title 5, § 4553(2)(D).

MARYLAND

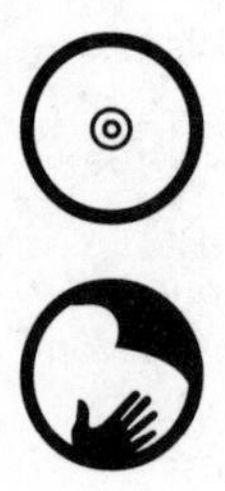

BREASTFEEDING

You can breastfeed your child anywhere that you are allowed to be.[1]

PREGNANCY

Your employer can't discriminate against you because of your sex.[2]

This law applies to employers who have fifteen or more employees.[3]

The law seems to also ban pregnancy discrimination.[4]

Maryland law also explicitly states that disabilities related to pregnancy are temporary disabilities and have to be treated as such under employer plans, such as sick leave. Disability due to pregnancy has to be treated the same as other temporary disabilities. [5]

Employers must provide reasonable accommodations upon an employee's request for employee's disability caused or contributed to by pregnancy, provided the accommodation does not impose an undue hardship on the employer. The employer must explore with the employee all possible means of providing the reasonable accommodation, including changing the employee's job duties, changing the employee's work hours, relocating the employee's work area, providing mechanical or electrical aids, transferring the employee to a less strenuous or

[1]Md. Code, Health-Gen. § 20-801.
[2]Md. Code, State Gov't § 20-606.
[3]Md. Code, State Gov't § 20-601(d).
[4]See Ferdinand-Davenport v. Children's Guild, 742 F. Supp. 2d 772, 783 (D. Md. 2010).
[5]Md. Code Ann., State Gov't § 20-609.

less hazardous position for the duration of the pregnancy, or providing leave. The law applies to employers with fifteen or more employees. The law went into effect October 1, 2013.[6] The Maryland Commission on Civil Rights clarified that this law applies not only to pregnancy-related disabilities, but to all pregnant employees.[7]

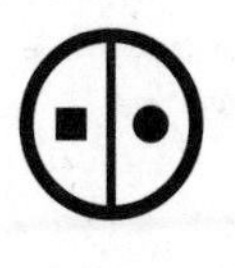

CAREGIVER DISCRIMINATION

A few localities in Maryland have laws that protect caregivers from discrimination, such as Cumberland.[8] For a complete list of Maryland localities' caregiver discrimination laws, check out http://www.worklifelaw.org/pubs/LocalFRDLawsDetail.html.

KINCARE

Employees in Maryland who work for employers with fifteen or more employees can use their own paid time off to care for immediate family members who are ill.[9]

PUBLIC-SECTOR WORKERS

As a government employee, you may be entitled to different benefits. Be sure to check your employee handbook or union contract or talk with human resources.

[6]Md. Code Ann. State Gov't § 20-609.

[7]"House Bill 804, amending § 20-606: (1) Requires that employers, upon request, explore all possible means of providing a reasonable accommodation to a pregnant employee, regardless of whether they do so with other employees who are temporarily disabled. (2) This applies to all pregnant employees who request an accommodation, not just women with pregnancy-related conditions/disabilities. However the employee may be required to provide a doctor's note." Email exchange between Glendora C. Hughes, General Counsel of the Maryland Commission on Civil Rights, and Liz Reiner Platt (Jan. 22, 2014, 17:07, 17:12 EST) (on file with author).

[8]Cumberland, Md. Code §§ 9-26 to -30.

[9]Md. Code, Lab. & Empl. § 3-802.

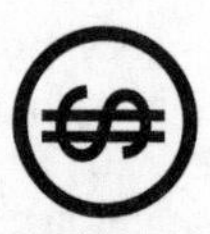

EQUAL PAY
Employers cannot discriminate on the basis of sex in paying employees in the same establishment.[10]

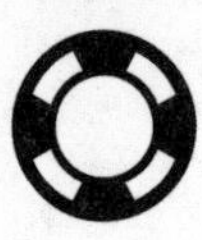

UNEMPLOYMENT INSURANCE
Maryland has a law stating that if you left work for a really compelling reason, then you might still be eligible for benefits, and it specifies that if you left to care for someone, you need to have evidence of a health problem from a hospital or physician.[11]

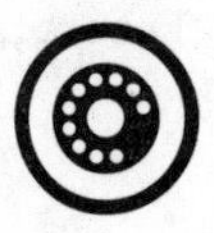

CALL FOR HELP
For questions about the law or to file a complaint, you may contact the Maryland Commission on Civil Rights:

Phone: 410-767-8600 / TTD: 410-333-1737
Address:
6 Saint Paul Street
Baltimore, MD 21202
Website: mccr.maryland.gov

[10]Md. Code, Lab. & Empl. § 3-304.
[11]Md. Code, Lab. & Empl. § 8-1001(c)(ii); 8-1001(c)(2).

MASSACHUSETTS

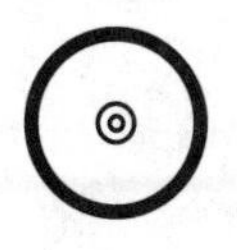

BREASTFEEDING

Mothers may breastfeed in places open to the general public, not including churches and other houses of worship or religious instruction.[1]

UNPAID FAMILY LEAVE

In addition to FMLA leave covering employers with fifty or more employees, Massachusetts has a law that applies to most employers with six or more employees[2] covering women who have worked full-time for the same employer for at least three months in a row (or those who have completed a probationary period) and providing up to eight weeks of maternity leave to give birth or adopt a child.[3] You have to give at least two weeks' notice to your employer.[4]

[1]Mass. Gen. Laws c. 111, § 221.
[2]Mass. Gen. Laws c. 151B, § 1(5).
[3]Mass. Gen. Laws c. 149, § 105D.
[4]Ibid. An interesting guideline issued by the Massachusetts Commission against Discrimination states that women who give birth to multiples get eight weeks per child, so a woman giving birth to twins (or adopting twins) gets sixteen weeks off, not just eight (http://www.mass.gov/mcad/maternity3.html). This isn't in the statute, just the agency guidance, so we caution you to consult with an attorney if you are having multiples and are interested in this right.

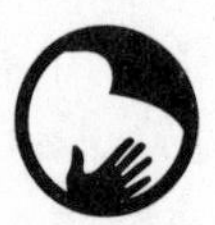

PREGNANCY

Massachusetts prohibits discrimination on the basis of sex;[5] the law applies to most employers with six or more employees.[6]

The prohibition includes pregnancy discrimination.[7]

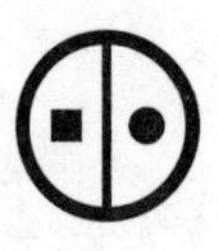

CAREGIVER DISCRIMINATION

In Boston it is illegal for employers to discriminate against parents.[8]

There are other localities in Massachusetts that provide protections as well; check out this website for the list: http://www.worklifelaw.org/pubs/LocalFRDLawsDetail.html.

PARENTAL INVOLVEMENT IN CHILDREN'S EDUCATION

You can take up to twenty-four hours of leave per year to participate in your child's school activities; if your leave is foreseeable, then you have to give seven days' notice to your employer.[9]

However, this right is only available to employees who work in companies of fifty or more and have worked for a year (i.e., you must meet the requirements of the FMLA).

PUBLIC-SECTOR WORKERS

As a government employee, you may be entitled to different benefits. Be sure to check your employee handbook or union contract or talk with human resources.

[5]Mass. Gen. Laws c. 151B, § 4.
[6]Mass. Gen. Laws c. 151B, § 1(5). Even if an employer has fewer than six employees, an employee could still possibly bring a successful suit under the Massachusetts Equal Rights Act. Thurdin v. SEI Boston, LLC, 895 N.E.2d 446 (Mass. 2008).
[7]See, for example, Mass. Elec. Co. v. Mass. Comm'n against Discrimination, 375 N.E.2d 1192 (Mass. 1978).
[8]Boston, Mass. Code § 12-9.3.
[9]Mass. Gen. Laws c. 149, § 52D(b)(1).

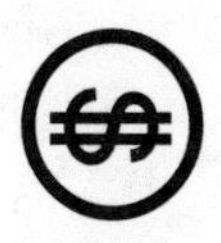

EQUAL PAY

Employers have to pay equal wages for men and women doing comparable work, unless the difference is based on seniority.[10]

OTHER

Massachusetts law lets you take time for taking your child to routine medical and dental appointments.[11]

However, this right is only available to employees who work in companies of fifty or more and have worked for a year (i.e., you must meet the requirements of the FMLA).

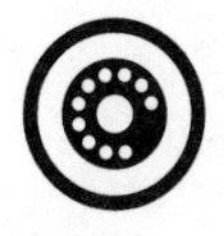

CALL FOR HELP

For more information about the law or to file a complaint, you may contact the Massachusetts Commission against Discrimination:

Phone:
Boston Office: 617-994-6000
Springfield Office: 413-739-2145
Worcester Office: 508-799-8010
New Bedford Office: 508-990-2390
Website: www.mass.gov/mcad

[10]Mass. Gen. Laws c. 149, § 105A.
[11]Mass. Gen. Laws c. 149, § 52D(b)(2).

MICHIGAN

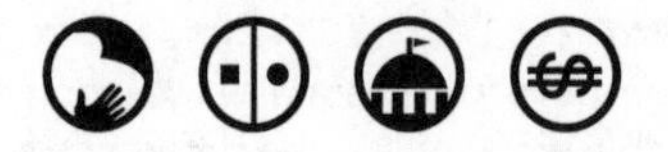

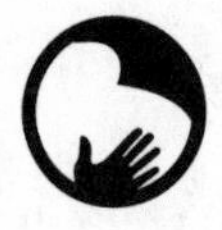

PREGNANCY

The Elliot-Larsen Civil Rights Act applies to all employers[1] and prohibits sex discrimination.[2] "Sex" is defined to include pregnancy and childbirth.[3]

The law also indicates that employers can't treat pregnant women any differently from other temporarily disabled workers who are similarly situated.[4]

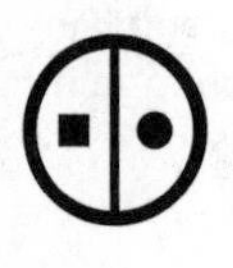

CAREGIVER DISCRIMINATION

There are a few different localities that provide some protections based on family status, such as Ann Arbor, which prohibits employers from discriminating on the basis of family responsibilities.[5] For a complete listing, view http://www.worklifelaw.org/pubs/LocalFRDLawsDetail.html.

PUBLIC-SECTOR WORKERS

As a government employee, you may be entitled to different benefits. Be sure to check your employee handbook or union contract or talk with human resources.

[1]Mich. Comp. Laws § 37.2201(a).
[2]Mich. Comp. Laws § 37.2202(1).
[3]Mich. Comp. Laws § 37.2201(d).
[4]Mich. Comp. Laws § 37.2202(1)(d). The law says an employer cannot: "Treat an individual affected by pregnancy, childbirth, or a related medical condition differently for any employment-related purpose from another individual who is not so affected but similar in ability or inability to work, without regard to the source of any condition affecting the other individual's ability or inability to work." This could be interpreted to mean that employers cannot make a distinction between pregnancy/childbirth limitations and on-the-job injuries—check with a Michigan lawyer to understand how this law plays out in practice.
[5]Ann Arbor, Mich. Code §§ 9:151(4); 9:154.

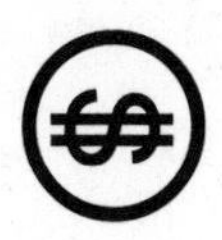

EQUAL PAY

Employers can't discriminate in wages between the sexes.[6]

Employers also can't discipline or discriminate against you because you disclosed your wages.[7]

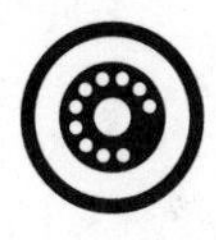

CALL FOR HELP

For questions about the law or to file a complaint, you may contact the Michigan Department of Civil Rights:

Phone: 800-482-3604
Address:
Capitol Tower Building
110 W. Michigan Avenue, Suite 800
Lansing, MI 48933
Website: www.michigan.gov/mdcr
Email: MDCR-INFO@michigan.gov

Other resources:

Mothering Justice
Website: www.motheringjustice.org

[6]Mich. Comp. Laws § 750.556.
[7]Mich. Comp. Laws § 408.483a.

MINNESOTA

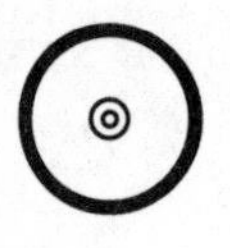

BREASTFEEDING

You can breastfeed your child anywhere you have a right to be.[1]

Employers have to give you breaks for expressing breast milk at work, and they have to try to find you a private space for pumping, other than a bathroom, with access to an electrical outlet.[2]

UNPAID FAMILY LEAVE

In addition to FMLA leave for employees working for employers with fifty or more workers, Minnesota law covers employees who have worked at least half-time at the same place for the last year[3] and applies to all employers with twenty-one or more employees.[4] Employers have to provide up to twelve weeks for an adoption or birth of a child, prenatal care, or for incapacity because of pregnancy, childbirth, or related health conditions.[5] While you are on leave, your employer has to continue to make insurance coverage available (but doesn't necessarily have to pay for it).[6]

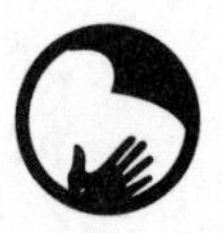

PREGNANCY

Employers can't discriminate against you on the basis of sex.[7] Sex is defined to include pregnancy and childbirth.[8] The law applies to most employers with one or more employees.[9]

[1]Minn. Stat. § 145.905.
[2]Minn. Stat. § 181.939.
[3]Minn. Stat. § 181.940(2).
[4]Minn. Stat. § 181.940(3).
[5]Minn. Stat. § 181.941(1).
[6]Minn. Stat. § 181.941(4).
[7]Minn. Stat. § 363A.08.
[8]Minn. Stat. § 363A.03(42).
[9]Minn. Stat. § 363A.03(16). See exceptions here: Minn. Stat. § 363A.20.

Minnesota law also requires employers to provide reasonable accommodations to employees for health conditions related to pregnancy or childbirth, unless it would impose an undue hardship.[10]

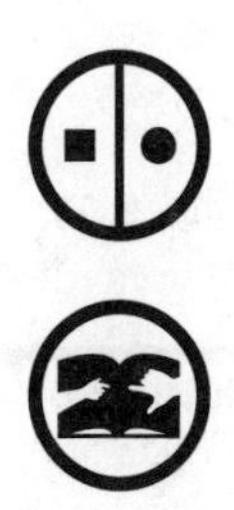

CAREGIVER DISCRIMINATION

Employers cannot discriminate against you because of your familial status, meaning that you are a parent or a legal guardian of a minor.[11]

PARENTAL INVOLVEMENT IN CHILDREN'S EDUCATION

Employers have to give you up to sixteen hours per year for school-related activities for your children–you have to give notice when you can.[12]

Take a look at the "Unpaid Family Leave" section; this law is under that statute's umbrella, although this particular provision applies to all employers with one or more employees.[13]

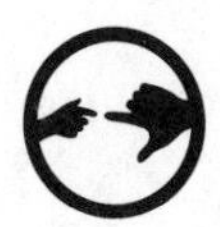

KINCARE

You can use your sick leave to care for your sick or injured child (now defined to include biological, adopted, foster, and stepchildren). Or for a sick or injured spouse, sibling, parent, grandparent, stepparent, mother-in-law, father-in-law, or grandchild (including step-grandchildren, adopted, and foster grandchildren).[14] Take a look at the Unpaid Family Leave section for some more specifics.

PUBLIC-SECTOR WORKERS

As a government employee, you may be entitled to different benefits. Be sure to check your employee handbook or union contract or talk with human resources.

[10]Minn. Stat. § 181.9414

[11]Minn. Stat. § 363A.08; Minn. Stat. §363A.03(18).

[12]Minn. Stat. § 181.9412.

[13]Minn. Stat. § 181.940(3).

[14]Minn. Stat. § 181.9413.

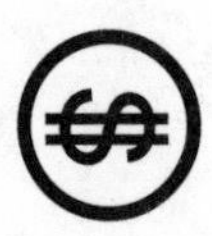

EQUAL PAY

Employers can't discriminate on the basis of sex in terms of wages.[15]

Employers cannot punish you for discussing your wages or require you to nondisclosure of your wages.[16]

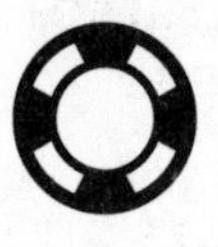

UNEMPLOYMENT INSURANCE

You might still be eligible for unemployment benefits if you quit in order to care for a sick, injured, or disabled immediate member of your family[17] or because your child care fell through.[18] In both cases you have to try to fix the situation (by asking your employer for an accommodation and trying to find other child care).

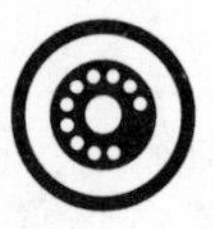

CALL FOR HELP

For questions about the law or to file a complaint, you may contact the Minnesota Department of Human Rights:

Phone: 651-539-1100 / TTY: 651-296-1283
Address:
Freeman Building
625 Robert Street North
Saint Paul, MN 55155
Website: www.humanrights.state.mn.us

Other resources:

Gender Justice
Phone: 651-789-2090
Website: www.genderjustice.us

[15]Minn. Stat. § 181.67.
[16]Minn. Stat. § 181.172.
[17]Minn. Stat. § 268.095(7)(ii).
[18]Minn. Stat. § 268.095(8).

MISSISSIPPI

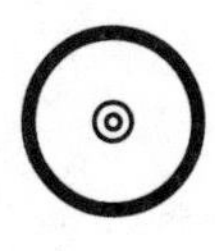

BREASTFEEDING

Mothers have a right to breastfeed wherever they are authorized to be.[1]

You also have a right to breastfeed your child or express milk at a licensed child care facility (including if you work there). They have to provide you with an outlet, a chair, access to running water, and a refrigerator.[2]

Your employer can't stop you from pumping breast milk during any break time.[3]

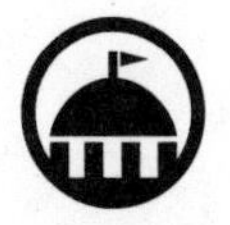

PUBLIC-SECTOR WORKERS

As a government employee, you may be entitled to different benefits. Be sure to check your employee handbook or union contract or talk with human resources.

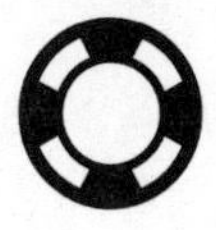

UNEMPLOYMENT INSURANCE

The law here is a bit complicated, but it says that if you leave work for marital or domestic reasons, then you can't get unemployment, but it also specifies that pregnancy is not considered a domestic reason, leaving the door open for getting benefits if you left because of pregnancy.[4] Be sure to consult with an attorney about this one.

[1]Miss. Code § 17-25-9.
[2]Miss. Code § 43-20-31.
[3]Miss. Code § 71-1-55.
[4]Miss. Code § 71-5-513(A)(1)(a).

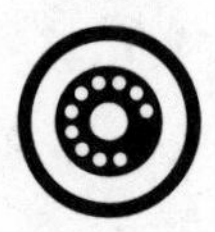

CALL FOR HELP

For questions about the state breastfeeding law, you may contact the Mississippi State Department of Health:

Address:
570 East Woodrow Wilson Drive
Jackson, MS 39216
Website: msdh.ms.gov

MISSOURI

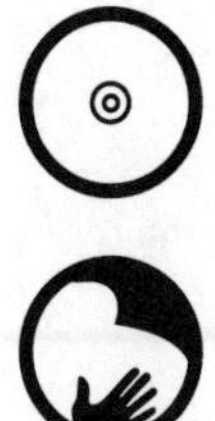

BREASTFEEDING

You can breastfeed your child anywhere you have a right to be.[1]

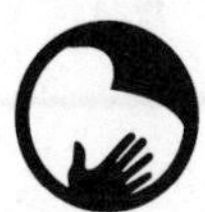

PREGNANCY

Employers can't discriminate against you on the basis of sex,[2] which seems to include pregnancy.[3] The law applies to employers with six or more employees (excluding religious corporations or associations).[4]

PUBLIC-SECTOR WORKERS

As a government employee, you may be entitled to different benefits. Be sure to check your employee handbook or union contract or talk with human resources.

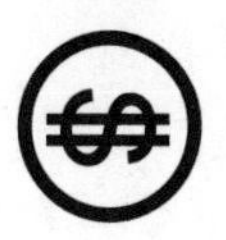

EQUAL PAY

Employers can't pay women less in wages than men unless the difference is based on something other than the sex of the employee.[5]

[1] Mo. Stat. § 191.918.
[2] Mo. Stat. § 213.055.
[3] See Self v. Midwest Orthopedics Foot & Ankle, P.C., 272 S.W.3d 364, 366 (Mo. Ct. App. 2008); see also Wierman v. Casey's General Stores, 638 F.3d 984, 1002 (8th Cir. 2011).
[4] Mo. Stat. § 213.010(7).
[5] Mo. Stat. § 290.410.

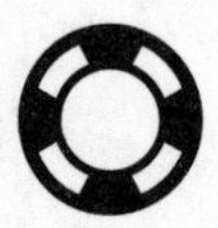

UNEMPLOYMENT INSURANCE

If you are forced to leave work due to pregnancy, then you might still be able to get benefits–there are requirements under the law (such as having medical documentation and having worked for the same employer for the last year), so take a careful look.[6]

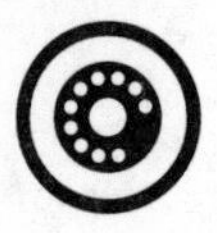

CALL FOR HELP

For questions about the law or to file a complaint, you may contact the Missouri Commission on Human Rights:

Phone: 877-781-4236 / TDD: 800-735-2966
Website: www.labor.mo.gov/mohumanrights

[6]Mo. Stat. § 288.050(1)(1)(d).

MONTANA

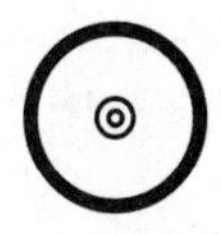

BREASTFEEDING

You have the right to breastfeed your child in any public or private place where you have the right to be,[1] but unless you work for the state or local government, you are not guaranteed time and space to express milk at work.

UNPAID FAMILY LEAVE

Montana has a maternity leave law that applies to employers of any size and protects you regardless of your tenure and number of hours you have worked.[2] As a birth mother, you are entitled to a reasonable leave of absence for pregnancy and childbirth,[3] which is usually about six to eight weeks for a normal pregnancy and delivery. You may be entitled to more time if you can't work before giving birth, or if you experience complications connected to your delivery. Your employer has to rely on the opinion of your doctor in determining what is a reasonable leave.[4]

You are entitled to have your job back (or an equivalent position) when you return from your pregnancy-related leave, unless it is impossible or unreasonable for your employer to do that.[5]

Your employer cannot force you to take maternity leave for an unreasonable period of time.[6]

[1]Mont. Code § 50-19-501.
[2]Mont. Code §§ 49-2-101(10)-(11), 49-2-310, 49-2-311.
[3]Mont. Code § 49-2-310(2).
[4]"Legal Rights of Pregnant Employees," Montana Department of Labor and Industry, Employment Relations Division, accessed January 11, 2013, http://erd.dli.mt.gov/human-rights/montana-human-rights-laws/employment-discrimination/rights-of-pregnant-employees.html.
[5]Mont. Code § 49-2-311.
[6]Mont. Code § 49-2-310(4).

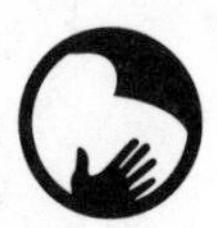

PREGNANCY

Montana state law prohibits discrimination based on sex and pregnancy in employment and applies to all employers regardless of size.[7]

You may be entitled to some workplace alterations to accommodate your pregnancy under Montana law as interpreted by the Montana Human Rights Bureau.[8]

Additionally, employers in Montana have a duty to provide all their employees with seats to use when not engaged in "active duties."[9]

PUBLIC-SECTOR WORKERS

As a government employee you may be entitled to additional benefits, such as leave for birth fathers and adoptive parents,[10] or unpaid break time to express milk for your baby.[11] Be sure to check your employee handbook or union contract or talk with human resources.

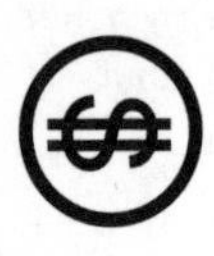

EQUAL PAY

The State of Montana has a stand-alone equal pay law that prohibits all employers from paying women less than men for equivalent service.[12]

The state, as an employer, is also working to establish a standard of equal pay for comparable worth.[13]

[7]Mont. Code §§ 49-2-303, 49-2-310(1).
[8]Mont. Code § 39-2-201.
[9]See, for example, Hauk v. Wal-Mart Stores, Human Rights Act Case No. 9801008431 (March 18, 1999), http://erd.dli.mt.gov/component/docman/doc_download/3787-hauk-v-wal-mart-.html; Auchenbach v. Community Nursing, Inc., Case No. 9401006303 (October 15, 1996), http://erd.dli.mt.gov/component/docman/doc_download/3822-auchenbach-v-community-nursing-.html.
[10]Mont. Code § 2-18-606.
[11]Mont. Code §§ 39-2-215 to 39-2-217.
[12]Mont. Code § 39-3-104.
[13]Mont. Code § 2-18-208.

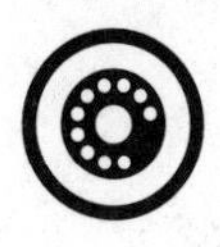

CALL FOR HELP

For questions and concerns about discrimination at work based on sex, pregnancy, or any other protected category, for questions about maternity leave, and to file a complaint, you may contact the Montana Human Rights Bureau:

Phone: 406-444-4356
Website: erd.dli.mt.gov/human-rights-bureau.html

NEBRASKA

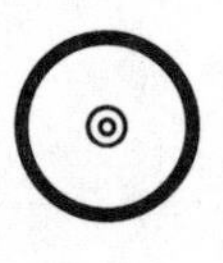

BREASTFEEDING

Although you may breastfeed your child in any public or private location where you are otherwise authorized to be,[1] there is no state law explicitly protecting your right to express breast milk at work.

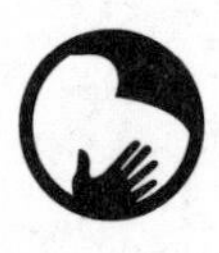

PREGNANCY

The Nebraska Fair Employment Practice Act covers employers with fifteen or more employees and prohibits discrimination on the basis of race, color, religion, age, sex (including pregnancy, childbirth, and related medical conditions), marital status, and national origin.[2]

State law also requires that pregnant women and those affected by childbirth or related conditions be treated the same as other workers similarly unable to work.[3]

If you work in academia, you may have extra protections under state law, which prohibits discrimination by educational institutions on the basis of sex in any program or activity. This includes discrimination on the basis of pregnancy and on parental status.[4]

[1]Neb. Rev. Stat. § 20-170.
[2]Neb. Rev. Stat. §§ 48-1104, 48-1102(13).
[3]Neb. Rev. Stat. § 48-1111.
[4]Neb. Rev. Stat. § 85-9,168.

PUBLIC-SECTOR WORKERS
As a state employee you may be entitled to request an alternative or flexible work schedule or to use your sick time to care for an immediate family member, among other benefits, so be sure to check your employee handbook or union contract or talk with human resources.[5]

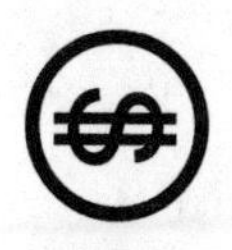

EQUAL PAY
Nebraska has a stand-alone state law prohibiting discrimination in pay based on sex.[6]

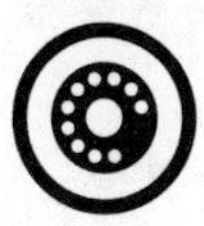

CALL FOR HELP
For questions about discrimination in employment based on sex, pregnancy, and other protected classes, you may contact the Nebraska Equal Opportunity Commission:

Phone: 402-471-2024
Address:
Nebraska State Office Building
301 Centennial Mall South, 5th Floor
Lincoln, NE 68509-4934

[5] See, for example, Human Resources Policy and Procedures Manual (Nebraska Administrative Services, created January 2002, revised March 2009), http://www.das.state.ne.us/personnel/hrcentral/as_hr_policy_and_procedure_manual.pdf.
[6] Neb. Rev. Stat. §§ 48-1219 to 48-1227.

NEVADA

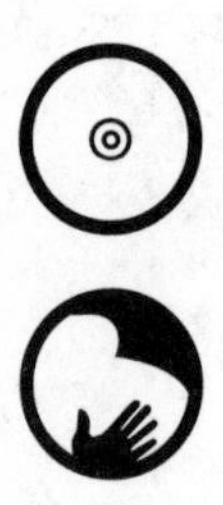

BREASTFEEDING

A mother may breastfeed her child in any public or private location where the mother is otherwise authorized to be.[1]

PREGNANCY

Nevada law prohibits employment discrimination on the basis of sex and based on pregnancy, childbirth, or related medical conditions.[2]

The law covers employers with fifteen or more employees.[3]

If your employer grants to your coworkers leave with or without pay, or leave without loss of seniority for sickness or disability because of a medical condition, it has to extend the same benefits to you as a pregnant woman. If you are entitled to leave as part of your employment benefits, you must be allowed to use that leave before and after childbirth, miscarriage, or other natural resolution of your pregnancy.[4]

PARENTAL INVOLVEMENT IN CHILDREN'S EDUCATION

Employers with fifty or more employees must grant employees up to four hours of unpaid leave per school year for each child enrolled in school, to attend certain school-related activities.[5]

No matter how small your employer, it may not terminate, demote, suspend, or discriminate against you for attend-

[1]Nev. Rev. Stat. § 201.232.
[2]Nev. Rev. Stat. § 613.330; Facts about Pregnancy Discrimination (Nevada Equal Rights Commission), http://detr.state.nv.us/nerc_pages/NERC_docs/Facts_About_Pregnancy_Discrimination.pdf.
[3]Nev. Rev. Stat. § 613.310.
[4]Nev. Rev. Stat. § 613.335.
[5]Nev. Rev. Stat. § 392.4577.

ing school conferences at the request of your child's school administrator or for leaving work when notified of a child's emergency.[6]

PUBLIC-SECTOR WORKERS

As a government employee, you may be eligible for sick leave to care for family members,[7] among other benefits, so be sure to check your employee handbook or union contract or talk with human resources.

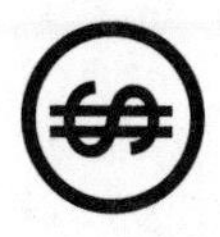

EQUAL PAY

Nevada explicitly prohibits paying men and women unequal wages for the same work.[8] This could include a neutral policy that has a negative impact on women–for example, providing extra compensation to employees who are the "head of household" (i.e., married with dependents and the primary financial contributor to the household).[9]

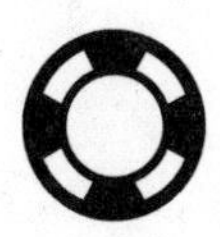

UNEMPLOYMENT INSURANCE

If you lose your job due to providing care for an immediate family member (spouse, parent, domestic partner, grandparent, sibling, or child) who is ill or has a disability, you may still be eligible for unemployment benefits.[10]

[6] Nev. Rev. Stat. § 392.920.

[7] See State of Nevada Employee Handbook (Department of Administration, Division of Human Resource Management), 19, http://dop.nv.gov/emphand.pdf.

[8] Nev. Rev. Stat. § 608.017(1).

[9] Equal Pay and Compensation Discrimination (Nevada Equal Rights Commission), http://detr.state.nv.us/nerc_pages/NERC_docs/Facts_About_Equal_Pay.pdf.

[10] Letter from Cynthia Jones, Deputy Director, Nevada Department of Employment, Training and Rehabilitation, to Cheryl Atkinson, Administrator, US Department of Labor (May 2009), retrieved October 11, 2011, from http://www.doleta.gov/recovery/pdf/NV2-3.pdf.

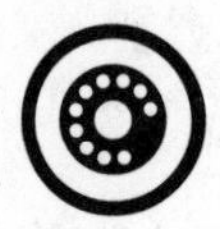

CALL FOR HELP

For information about the law and help with problems at work regarding your pregnancy or sex discrimination, you may contact the Nevada Equal Rights Commission:

Phone: 702-486-7161
Address:
1820 East Sahara Avenue, Suite 314
Las Vegas, NV 89104
Fax: 702-486-7054
Website: www.detr.state.nv.us

NEW HAMPSHIRE

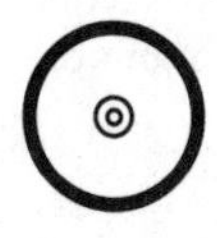

BREASTFEEDING

As a nursing mother, you are protected, broadly, from discrimination in the form of any limit or restriction on your right to breastfeed.[1]

That could include discrimination against you for feeding your baby in a restaurant or discrimination by your employer because you want to pump milk at work.

UNPAID FAMILY LEAVE

See Pregnancy section.

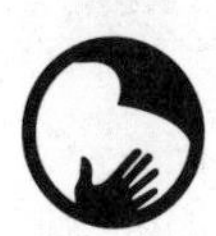

PREGNANCY

If your employer has six or more employees, you are protected from discrimination because of pregnancy or because of any medical condition resulting from pregnancy.[2]

You are entitled to job-protected leave while you are physically unable to work because of pregnancy, childbirth, or a related medical condition. That means you can take the time you need when suffering from morning sickness and the time you need to recover from giving birth without worrying about losing your job. Your employer has to keep your original job or a comparable one open for you, unless business necessity makes this impossible or unreasonable.[3]

Your employer must provide the same benefits to you while you are on pregnancy-related leave as it does for coworkers on disability leave.[4]

[1] N.H. Rev. Stat. § 132:10-d.
[2] N.H. Rev. Stat. § 354-A:7(VI)(a).
[3] N.H. Rev. Stat. § 354-A:2(VI)-(VII), 354-A:7(VI)(b).
[4] N.H. Rev. Stat. § 354-A:7(VI)(c).

According to the executive director for the New Hampshire Commission for Human Rights, some conditions of pregnancy that may not qualify as a "disability"–such as a tipped uterus–must nevertheless be accommodated under New Hampshire pregnancy discrimination law.[5] A worker with such a condition must bring in a doctor's note documenting the accommodation she needs.

PUBLIC-SECTOR WORKERS

As a government employee, you may be entitled to more generous benefits, such as paid sick time or access to temporary disability insurance when you are on maternity leave. Be sure to check your employee handbook or union contract or talk with human resources.

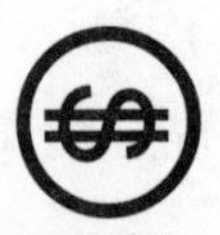

EQUAL PAY

New Hampshire state law outlaws discrimination in pay based on sex.[6]

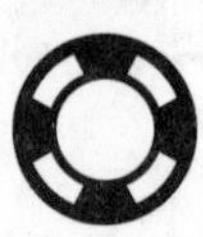

UNEMPLOYMENT INSURANCE

If you lose your job due to illness or disability of an immediate family member, you can still be eligible for unemployment benefits.[7]

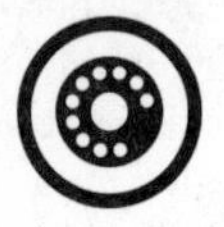

CALL FOR HELP

For questions about discrimination at work based on sex, pregnancy, disability, marital status, or any other protected category, contact New Hampshire Commission on Human Rights:

Phone: 603-271-2767
Address:
2 Chenell Drive, Unit 2
Concord, NH 03301-8501
Email: humanrights@nhsa.state.nh.us
Website:www.nh.gov/hrc/index.html

[5]Telephone conversation with Joni Esperian, Executive Director, New Hampshire Commission for Human Rights, (Dec. 17, 2013).

[6]N.H. Rev. Stat § 275:37.

[7]N.H. Rev. Stat. § 282-A:32(I)(a)(6).

NEW JERSEY

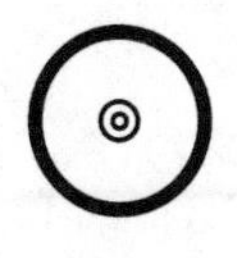

BREASTFEEDING

Although you are entitled to breastfeed in public in New Jersey,[1] there is no state law that explicitly protects your right to breastfeed or express milk at work.

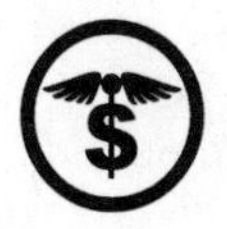

TEMPORARY DISABILITY INSURANCE

As a pregnant woman in New Jersey, you are likely eligible for temporary disability insurance benefits to cover your lost pay when you are unable to work because of pregnancy or delivery of a child. (Certain government workers are excluded under the law, and you must meet certain wage requirements to be covered.)[2]

The benefit is calculated as two-thirds of your average weekly wage, up to a maximum of $595.00 per week (as of January 1, 2014).[3]

Typically, you may receive benefits for up to four weeks before your expected delivery date and up to six weeks after the actual delivery date. If your doctor orders you on bed rest while you are pregnant, or you suffer complications from delivery, you may be able to receive benefits for a longer period of time.[4]

[1] N.J. Stat. § 26:4B-4.

[2] N.J. Stat. §§ 43:21-25 to 43:21-31; see also "Frequently Asked Questions—New Jersey Temporary Disability Insurance," State of New Jersey, Department of Labor and Workforce Development, accessed January 11, 2013, http://lwd.dol.state.nj.us/labor/tdi/content/faq.html.

[3] "Calculating Benefit Amounts—State Plan," State of New Jersey, Department of Labor and Workforce Development, accessed January 11, 2013, http://lwd.dol.state.nj.us/labor/tdi/worker/state/sp_calculating_bene_amounts.html.

[4] "Frequently Asked Questions—New Jersey Temporary Disability Insurance."

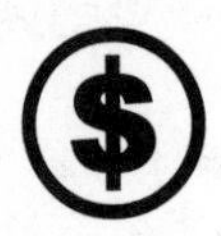

PAID FAMILY LEAVE

If you work in New Jersey, you are also likely eligible for family leave insurance, which provides some wage replacement for up to six weeks when you need to care for a family member who can't care for him or herself. Benefits are available (1) to bond with your child during the first twelve months after your child's birth or during the first twelve months after your child is placed with you for adoption and (2) to care for a family member with a serious health condition.[5]

The benefit is calculated as two-thirds of your average weekly wage, up to a maximum of $595.00 per week (as of January 1, 2014).[6]

UNPAID FAMILY LEAVE

New Jersey makes a modest addition to the job protection of the FMLA, providing job-protected leave if the New Jersey employer has fifty employees worldwide (rather than just in a seventy-five-mile radius) for those who have worked for that employer for at least twelve months and at least one thousand hours in the last twelve months. New Jersey also covers care for civil union partners, registered domestic partners, and same-sex spouses as well as other listed FMLA relatives.[7]

Unlike the FMLA, you cannot use the expanded New Jersey Family Leave to recover from your own illness or pregnancy-related disability. But the New Jersey Law Against Discrimination (which covers all employers, regardless of size) does protect you from unfair treatment at work related to your pregnancy or childbirth (including maternity leave).[8]

[5]N.J. Stat. §§ 43:21-39.1 to 43:21-39.3 (2012); see also Guide to New Jersey Family Leave Insurance (A Better Balance, February 2012), http://abetterbalance.org/web/images/stories/Documents/familyleave/general/NJFamilyLeaveGuide2012.pdf.

[6]"Benefit Calculation and Duration of Benefits," State of New Jersey, Department of Labor and Workforce Development, accessed January 11, 2013, http://lwd.dol.state.nj.us/labor/fli/worker/state/FL_SP_calculating_benefits.html.

[7]N.J. Stat. § 34:11B-3.

[8]N.J. Stat. § 10:5-5, 10:5-12; Fact Sheet: Pregnant Women and Discrimination—Your Rights (New Jersey Office of the Attorney General, Division on Civil Rights), http://www.state.nj.us/lps/dcr/downloads/fact_preg.pdf.

If your situation is covered by both the New Jersey Family Leave Act and the Family and Medical Leave Act (e.g., you need to care for an ailing spouse), you must take both types of leave at the same time. However, if you need to take time off for your own pregnancy-related disability (say, your doctor orders you onto bed rest for twelve weeks) and then need time to bond with a new child, you can use the FMLA and the NJFLA back-to-back and end up with as many as twenty-four total weeks of leave.

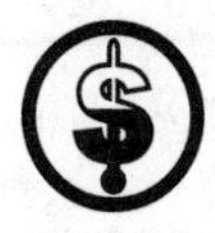

PAID SICK DAYS

In Jersey City, employers with ten or more employees must provide up to forty hours paid sick time per year, that workers can use for their own or a family member's health needs (like sickness or a check-up). Employers with fewer than ten employees must provide up to forty hours unpaid sick time. Workers earn one hour of sick time for every thirty hours worked.[9]

In Newark, people who work for any employer with ten or more employees–as well as all child care, home health care, and food service workers, regardless of the size of their employer–must receive up to forty hours paid sick time per year. Workers can use this time for their own or a family member's health needs. Employers with fewer than ten employees must provide up to twenty-four hours paid sick time. Workers earn one hour of sick time for every thirty hours worked.[10]

PREGNANCY

The New Jersey Law Against Discrimination covers employers regardless of size and all employees except domestic workers.[11]

[9]Jersey City, New Jersey Municipal Code § 3-50, et seq.

[10]Newark Municipal Council 13-2010 (N.J. 2014), available at: https://newark.legistar.com/LegislationDetail.aspx?ID=1518218&GUID=22C72D79-0A2C-4DF9-A597-9FF29C980CF6&Options=&Search=&FullText=1.

[11]N.J. Stat. § 10:5-5(e).

The law prohibits discrimination in employment based on sex, including pregnancy.[12]

In January 2014, New Jersey passed S2995/A4486,[13] which provides important new protections to pregnant workers. Now, your employer has to accommodate many needs at work that you have because of pregnancy, childbirth, or a related medical condition, if you ask for the accommodation based on the advice of your doctor. Your employer does not have to accommodate you if he or she can show that the accommodation would be an "undue hardship." Examples of accommodations that are covered by the New Jersey law include bathroom breaks, breaks to drink water, periodic rest, assistance with manual labor, job restructuring or modified work schedules, and temporary transfers to less strenuous or hazardous work. If your employer refuses to give you an accommodation, or punishes you for asking for or using an accommodation, this may be pregnancy discrimination so call a lawyer.

In addition, your employer cannot offer pregnant workers accommodations or leave in a way that is less favorable than accommodations or leave that is offered to non-pregnant workers who are similar in their inability or ability to work. For example: your boss cannot have a policy that offers two weeks leave for recovery from childbirth and four weeks leave for all other hospitalizations.

CAREGIVER DISCRIMINATION

If you work for the State of New Jersey, you are protected from discrimination at work based on your "familial status."[14] That includes discrimination against you by another state employee or by anyone doing business with the state. Several localities in

[12]N.J. Stat. §§ 10:5-3.1; 10:5-12(s); Fact Sheet: Pregnant Women & Discrimination—Your Rights.

[13]N.J. Stat. §§ 10:5-3.1; 10:5-12(s).

[14]N.J. Admin. Code § 4A:7-3.1.

New Jersey, including the cities of Newark and Passaic and the boroughs of Rocky Hill and Wanaque, have outlawed discrimination against city employees based on familial status or family responsibilities.[15]

PUBLIC-SECTOR WORKERS

As a government employee, you may be entitled to more generous benefits, such as paid sick time to care for family members.[16] Be sure to check your employee handbook or union contract or talk with human resources.

EQUAL PAY

New Jersey specifically prohibits discrimination in pay based on sex.[17]

In 2012, New Jersey enacted a law that prohibits employers from retaliating against employees for requesting or disclosing their compensation, benefits, or other personal information when they reasonably believe that there is a pay discrimination problem.[18]

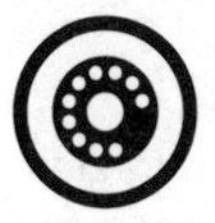

CALL FOR HELP

For questions about the New Jersey Family Leave Act or workplace discrimination or to file a complaint, contact the New Jersey Office of the Attorney General, Division of Civil Rights:

Website: www.NJCivilRights.gov.

For questions about New Jersey family leave insurance or temporary disability insurance, contact the New Jersey Department of Labor and Workforce Development:

Phone: 609-659-9045
Website: lwd.dol.state.nj.us/labor/index.html

[15]See Newark Code § 2:2-84.4; Passaic Code §§ 35-1 to 35-15; Rocky Hill Code § 24-9 to 24-20; Wanaque Code § 29-22 to 29-24.

[16]N.J. Admin. Code § 4A:6-1.3(g)(3).

[17]N.J. Stat. § 34:11-56.2.

[18]N.J. Stat. §§ 34:19-3(d); 10:5-12(r).

NEW MEXICO

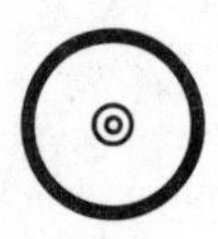

BREASTFEEDING

You may breastfeed your child in any public or private location where you are authorized to be.[1]

If you work for an employer with four or more employees, you are entitled to break time and a private space to express breast milk. Your employer must provide a clean, private place (not a bathroom) near your workspace for you to pump. They must also provide flexible breaks for you to pump, although they don't have to pay you for that time.[2]

PREGNANCY

If you work for an employer with four or more employees, the New Mexico Human Rights Act protects you from pregnancy discrimination. In addition, your employer has to treat you the same as your coworkers who are temporarily disabled. This includes equal access to benefits.[3]

PUBLIC-SECTOR WORKERS

As a government employee, you may be entitled to more generous benefits, such as paid sick time to care for family members.[4] Be sure to check your employee handbook or union contract or talk with human resources.

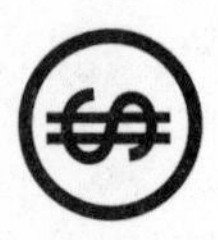

EQUAL PAY

Although the State of New Mexico does not have a stand-alone equal pay law, the Human Rights Act does prohibit employers with four or more employees from discriminating in compen-

[1] N.M. Stat. § 28-20-1.
[2] N.M. Stat. § 28-20-2.
[3] See N.M. Code R. § 9.1.1.7 (HH) (2).
[4] See N.M. Code R. § 1.7.7.10 (D).

sation based on sex. Also, the state has a policy of pay equity and requires those doing business with it (i.e., state contractors) to submit gender pay equity reports.[5]

The New Mexico Fair Pay for Women Act prohibits employers with four or more employees from engaging in wage discrimination on the basis of sex in the same establishment for equal work on jobs that require equal skill, effort, and responsibility and that are performed under similar working conditions, except where the payment is made pursuant to a seniority system, merit system, or system that measures earnings by quantity or quality of production. The law also protects employees against retaliation.[6]

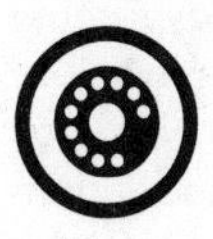

CALL FOR HELP

For questions or concerns about discrimination at work based on sex, pregnancy, or any other protected category, contact the New Mexico Department of Workforce Solutions, Human Rights Bureau:

Phone: 505-827-6838
Address:
1596 Pacheco Street, Suite 103
Santa Fe, NM 87505

[5]N.M. Stat. § 28-1-2, 28-1-7(A).
[6]New Mexico Pay Equity Initiative, Executive Order Number 2009-049: Frequently Asked Questions (January 20, 2010), http://www.generalservices.state.nm.us/uploads/ FileLinks/864df4748b2440569b3af8a95ce155d8/ContractorFAQs.pdf.
[7]N.M. Stat. § 28-23-3.

NEW YORK

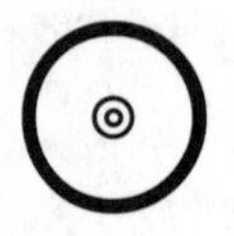

BREASTFEEDING

You are free to breastfeed your child in any public or private location where you have the right to be.[1]

Your employer, no matter its size, must give you unpaid break time to express breast milk at work (or allow you to pump during regularly scheduled paid breaks). Your employer must also make a reasonable attempt to provide a private location, other than a bathroom, for you to express milk. Finally, your employer may not discriminate against you for choosing to express milk at work.[2]

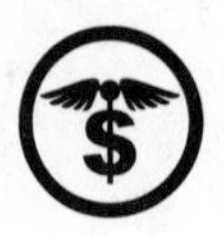

TEMPORARY DISABILITY INSURANCE

As a pregnant woman, you are likely eligible for temporary disability insurance benefits to cover your lost pay when you are unable to work because of pregnancy or delivery of a child. (Certain government workers are excluded under the law, and you must meet certain wage requirements to be covered.)[3]

New York's temporary disability insurance (TDI) program calculates benefits at 50 percent of your average weekly wage, up to a maximum of $170.00 per week.[4]

[1] N.Y. Civil Rights Law § 79-e.
[2] N.Y. Lab. Law § 206-c.
[3] N.Y. Workers' Comp. Law §§ 201-205.
[4] A Guide to Temporary Disability Benefits: Employee Benefits for Injuries and Illnesses That Occur Off the Job in New York (N.Y. State Workers' Compensation Board), 2, http://www.wcb.ny.gov/content/main/TheBoard/DB_BenefitGuide_P20.pdf.

Although workers are eligible for up to twenty-six weeks of TDI, the typical period of pregnancy-related disability is four to six weeks prior to a woman's due date and four to six weeks after delivery.[5]

The New York TDI law does not offer job protection while you are out on disability, but your employer is not allowed to retaliate against you for claiming or attempting to claim benefits.[6]

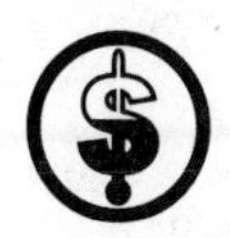

PAID SICK DAYS

If you are one of the 3.4 million private-sector workers in New York City, you are in luck! On April 1, 2014, the New York City Earned Sick Time Act went into effect. This landmark law ensures that workers in New York City can take time off for personal or family health needs without losing their jobs, and provides paid sick time to many of these workers. Here's an overview of what the law provides:[7]

- All private-sector workers, even those in the smallest businesses, cannot be fired or punished for taking up to forty hours of unpaid sick time per year.
- Private-sector workers in businesses with five or more employees will earn one hour of paid sick time for every thirty hours worked, and they will be able to earn up to forty hours of paid sick time per year. The law covers full-time, part-time, and most temporary workers.
- Domestic workers in New York City will be entitled to two paid sick days in addition to the "days of rest" they receive under state law.
- Paid or unpaid sick time can be used to care for a worker's own health needs or to care for the health needs of a worker's spouse, domestic partner, child, parent, grandparent, grandchild, sibling, or the child or parent of a worker's spouse or domestic partner.

[5] Ibid., 3.
[6] N.Y. Workers' Comp. Law § 241.
[7] N.Y.C. Admin. Code § 20-911 et seq.

– Any type of paid leave a worker already gets, such as paid vacation or personal days, will count for purposes of complying with the law as long as it can be used under the same conditions and for the same purposes as the Earned Sick Time Act.

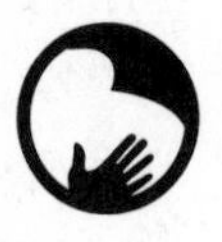

PREGNANCY[7]

New York law prohibits discrimination based on sex, which includes pregnancy, and covers employers with four or more employees.[8]

Under the law, an employer also may not force you to take a leave of absence during your pregnancy, unless your pregnancy prevents you from doing your job in a reasonable manner.[9]

New York City passed the Pregnant Workers Fairness Act in 2013. This law requires employers reasonably accommodate you if you have needs related to your pregnancy, birth, or a related medical condition. The law applies to full- and part-time workers, if your employer is located in NYC and has four or more employees. An employer does not have to accommodate you if doing so would be an "undue hardship." Examples of accommodations you may need include water or bathroom breaks, light duty, or time off to recover from childbirth.[10]

[8]You also may be able to seek a workplace accommodation to allow you to continue working while pregnant. For information about New York State law, check out http://www.dhr.ny.gov/sites/default/files/pdf/pregnancy.pdf. Legislation proposed by Governor Cuomo in January 2013, the Women's Equality Agenda, would, if passed, include explicit protections for pregnant women seeking workplace modifications to stay healthy and on the job, as well as enhanced equal pay and family status protections. See Governor Andrew M. Cuomo, NY Rising: 2013 State of the State, 115–26 (January 9, 2013), http://www.governor.ny.gov/sites/default/themes/governor/sos2013/2013SOSBook.pdf. Check our website, www.abetterbalance.org, for any updates on the bill.

[9]N.Y. Exec. Law § 296; see Mittl v. N.Y. State Div. of Human Rights, 794 N.E.2d 660 (N.Y. 2003) ("Article 15 of the Executive Law—known as the Human Rights Law—prohibits discharge of an employee because of pregnancy").

[10]N.Y. Exec. Law § 296(g).

CAREGIVER DISCRIMINATION

Ithaca, Rye Brook, and Westchester County have laws prohibiting employment discrimination based on familial status or parental status by public and/or private employers. Check this website to find out more: http://www.worklifelaw.org/pubs/LocalFRDLawsDetail.html.

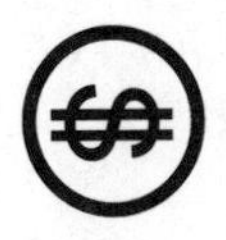

PUBLIC-SECTOR WORKERS

As a state employee, you may be entitled to more generous benefits, such as paid sick time to care for family members and up to seven months of unpaid leave following the birth or adoption of a child.[11] Be sure to check your employee handbook or union contract or talk with human resources.

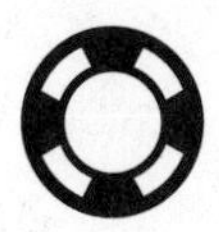

EQUAL PAY

New York has its own equal pay law, which prohibits employers from paying employees of different sexes different wages for equal work in the same establishment.[13]

UNEMPLOYMENT INSURANCE

As a New Yorker, if you lose your job due to illness or disability of an immediate family member, you may still be eligible for unemployment insurance.[14]

OTHER

If your employer (or the government agency where you work) permits employees to take leave upon the birth of a child, they must allow you, as an adoptive parent, to take the same leave on the same terms.[15]

[11]N.Y.C. Admin. Code § 8-107(22).
[12]New York State Department of Civil Service, "Leaves without Pay" (Part 22), Attendance and Leave Manual, Section 22.1.
[13]N.Y. Lab. Law § 194.
[14]N.Y. Lab. Law § 593(1)(b)(ii).
[15]N.Y. Lab. Law § 201-c.

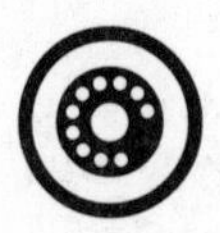

CALL FOR HELP

For questions about employment discrimination (including that based on sex, pregnancy, or marital status), you can contact the New York State Division of Human Rights:

Phone: 888-392-3644
Website: www.dhr.ny.gov

For questions about your workplace rights as a nursing mother and about other labor law issues, you can contact the New York Department of Labor:

Phone: 518-457-9000
Website: http://www.labor.ny.gov/home

If you work in New York, you can also contact us and our Families @ Work Legal Clinic, at 212-430-5982, regarding any questions about your workplace rights as an expecting or new parent.

NORTH CAROLINA

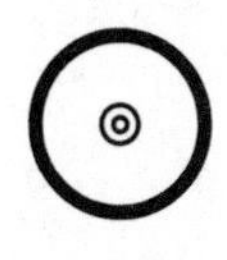

BREASTFEEDING
Although you have the right to breastfeed in any public or private location where you are otherwise authorized to be,[1] there is no state law that explicitly protects your right to breastfeed or express milk at work.

PARENTAL INVOLVEMENT IN CHILDREN'S EDUCATION
As a parent or guardian of a school-age child, you are entitled to four hours per year of unpaid leave to attend or otherwise be involved in your child's school. Your employer can't fire or demote you or take other negative action against you for requesting or taking the leave.[2]

PUBLIC-SECTOR WORKERS
As a government employee, you may be entitled to more generous benefits, such as paid sick time to care for family members, including an immediate family member who is disabled due to childbirth.[3] Be sure to check your employee handbook or union contract or talk with human resources.

[1]N.C. Gen. Stat. § 14-190.9(b).
[2]N.C. Gen. Stat. § 95-28.3.
[3]See *Inside North Carolina: A Guide to State Employment* (North Carolina Office of State Personnel, October 1, 2012), 39, http://www.osp.state.nc.us/State%20Employee%20Handbook%202012.pdf.

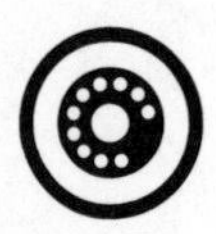

CALL FOR HELP

Even though North Carolina has no state employment discrimination laws, there is a state Human Relations Commission, which "serves as a clearinghouse to disseminate information concerning North Carolina's employment law to citizens." You can contact the North Carolina Human Relations Commission here:

Phone: 919-807-4420
Address:
116 W. Jones Street, Suite 2109
Raleigh, NC 27601

If you have questions about the state parental involvement law, you will have to consult with an attorney because the North Carolina Department of Labor does not administer the law.

NORTH DAKOTA

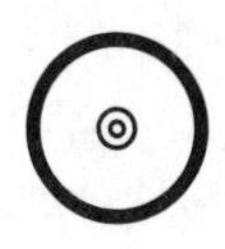

BREASTFEEDING

Although you have the right to breastfeed your child in any location, public or private, where you are otherwise authorized to be,[1] there is no state law that explicitly protects you as a nursing mom at work. The state does allow employers to call themselves "infant friendly" if they adopt certain workplace breastfeeding policies.[2]

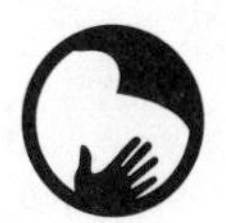

PREGNANCY

The North Dakota Human Rights Act makes it illegal for an employer with one or more employees to discriminate on the basis of sex, including pregnancy, childbirth, and related disabilities.[3]

PUBLIC-SECTOR WORKERS

As a state employee, you may be entitled to more generous benefits, such as leave to care for a spouse with a serious health condition.[4] Be sure to check your employee handbook or union contract or talk with human resources.

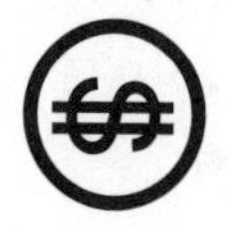

EQUAL PAY

North Dakota law forbids employers from paying unequal wages for comparable work to employees in the same workplace, based on their gender.[5]

[1]N.D. Cent. Code § 23-12-16.
[2]N.D. Cent. Code § 23-12-17.
[3]N.D. Cent. Code § 14-02.4.03.
[4]N.D. Cent. Code § 54-52.4-03.
[5]N.D. Cent. Code Chapter 34-06.1.03.

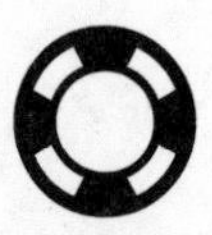

UNEMPLOYMENT INSURANCE
You may still be eligible for unemployment benefits in North Dakota even if you leave your job because of illness, disability, or need to care for a sick family member.[6]

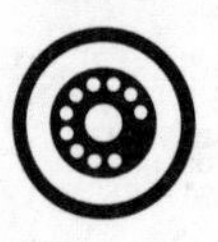

CALL FOR HELP
For questions about workplace discrimination or to file a complaint, you may contact the North Dakota Department of Labor, Human Rights Division:

Phone: 701-328-2660
Address:
600 East Boulevard Avenue, Dept. 406
Bismarck, ND 58505-0340
Email: humanrights@nd.gov
Website: www.nd.gov/labor/human-rights

[6]Rick McHugh et. al., *Between a Rock and a Hard Place: Confronting the Failure of State Unemployment Insurance Systems to Serve Women and Working Families* (National Employment Law Project, July 2003), 40, http://nelp.3cdn.net/ebba1e75e059fc749d_0um6idptk.pdf.

OHIO

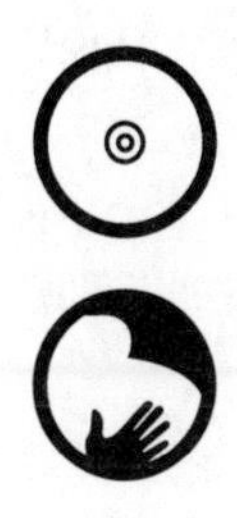

BREASTFEEDING

As a nursing mom, you are entitled to breastfeed your baby in any public place where you are otherwise permitted.[1]

PREGNANCY

Employers with four or more employees must not discriminate against women because of their sex, which includes pregnancy, childbirth, and related medical conditions.[2] However, the Supreme Court of Ohio recently found that state law does not require employers to provide a minimum amount of leave for pregnancy and childbirth.[3]

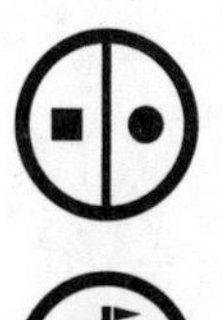

CAREGIVER DISCRIMINATION

The town of Xenia prohibits employers with four or more employees from discriminating based on familial status.[4]

PUBLIC-SECTOR WORKERS

As a state employee, you may be entitled to more generous benefits, such as paid and unpaid parental leave,[5] and sick time that can be used to care for ill family members.[6] Be sure to

[1]Ohio Rev. Code § 3781.55 (2005).

[2]Ohio Rev. Code §§ 4112.01(B), 4112.02.

[3]See *McFee v. Nursing Care Mgt. of Am., Inc.*, 931 N.E.2d 1069 (Ohio 2010) (holding that the Ohio Civil Rights Commission's administrative regulations do not and cannot impose a requirement on all employers to provide a reasonable amount of leave for pregnancy and maternity leave); see also *Ware v. Jenny Craig, Inc.*, No. 1:11-cv-252, 2011 WL 5506102 (S.D. Ohio 2011) ("As a matter of Ohio law, employers are not required to provide maternity leave to persons, such as plaintiff, who do not meet the minimum eligibility requirements for a job-protected leave of absence under their employer's policies or under the FMLA").

[4]Xenia, Ohio Code §§ 604.01, 620.01-620.99.

[5]Ohio Rev. Code § 124.136.

[6]Ohio Admin. Code §§ 123:1-32-05(A)(5) & (6), 123:1-47-01(A)(39).

check your employee handbook or union contract or talk with human resources.

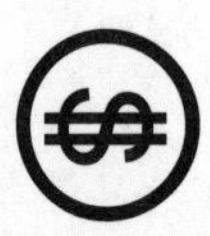

EQUAL PAY

Ohio law prohibits discriminatory pay practices based on race, color, religion, sex, age, national origin, or ancestry.[7]

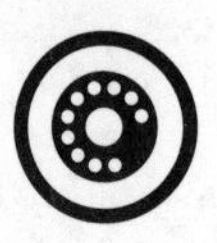

CALL FOR HELP

If you suspect discrimination or if you want to file a complaint, you may contact the Ohio Civil Rights Commission:

Phone: 888-278-7101
Website: crc.ohio.gov

[7]Ohio Rev. Code § 4111.17.

OKLAHOMA

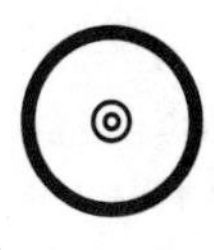

BREASTFEEDING

As a nursing mom, you have the right to breastfeed your child in any location where you are allowed to be.[1]

Oklahoma law allows employers to provide reasonable unpaid break time in an area other than a toilet stall for employees to pump breast milk or breastfeed their babies[2]—but note that this statute is worded in an odd way; it says employers may provide this but doesn't seem to require them to. Consult a lawyer about this confusing law.

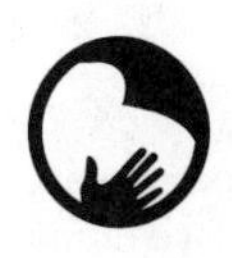

PREGNANCY

If you work for an employer with one or more employees (i.e., it could be just you), you are protected from discrimination in employment on the basis of sex, which includes pregnancy, childbirth, or related medical conditions.[3]

In some circumstances, pregnant women in Oklahoma may be entitled to reasonable accommodations at work. According to a memo from the Office of the Attorney General, workers with "pregnancy related disabilities and/or impairments and limitations" that fall within the statutory definition of a "disability" are eligible for accommodations, regardless of the "length or severity of the impairment."[4] This may be true even when there is no similarly-situated employee who has been accommodated, since it "is reasonable to believe that such accommodations be made in the absence of another employee in need of same or similar accommodations."

[1] Okla. Stat. title 63, § 1-234.1.
[2] Okla. Stat. title 40, § 435.
[3] Okla. Stat. title 25 § 1301 et seq.
[4] Memorandum from Candice Milard, Oklahoma Attorney General's Office (Feb. 13, 2014) (on file with author).

PUBLIC-SECTOR WORKERS

As a state employee, you may be entitled to more generous benefits, so be sure to check your employee handbook or union contract or talk with human resources.

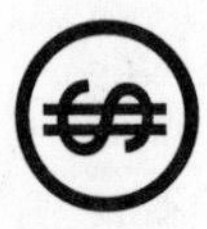

EQUAL PAY

Oklahoma forbids all employers from paying women less than men for comparable work.[5] The Commissioner of Labor is tasked with investigating potential violations of the law.[6]

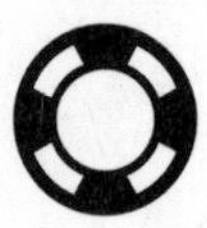

UNEMPLOYMENT INSURANCE

If you lose your job because of the illness or disability of an immediate family member (spouse, parent, or minor child), you may still be eligible for unemployment insurance under state law.[7]

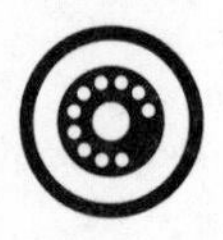

CALL FOR HELP

If you have questions about, or feel you may have experienced, discrimination on the job, you may contact the Oklahoma Attorney General's Office of Civil Rights Enforcement:

Phone: 405-521-2029
Email: OCRE@oag.ok.gov
Website: www.oag.state.ok.us/oagweb.nsf/ocre.html

[5]Okla. Stat. title 40 §198.1.
[6]Okla. Stat. title 40 §198.2.
[7]Okla. Stat. title 40 § 2-210.

OREGON

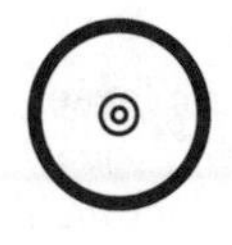

BREASTFEEDING

As a nursing mother, you have the right to breastfeed in public,[1] and if you work for an employer with twenty-five or more employees, you are entitled to reasonable unpaid rest periods (generally thirty minutes every four hours) to express breast milk while at work.[2] Employers are also required to make "reasonable efforts to provide a location, other than a public restroom or toilet stall, in close proximity to the employee's work area for the employee to express milk in private".[3]

UNPAID FAMILY LEAVE

The Oregon Family Leave Act (OFLA) guarantees up to twelve weeks, within a one-year period, of unpaid, job-protected family and medical leave to employees who work for employers with twenty-five or more employees in Oregon.[4] If eligible, you may use this leave for one of four purposes:

- to recover from or seek treatment for your own serious health condition (which includes pregnancy)
- to care for a family member (including a grandparent or grandchild, parent-in-law,[5] or domestic partner or child of a domestic partner[6]) with a serious health condition

[1]Or. Rev. Stat. § 109.001.
[2]Or. Rev. Stat. § 653.077; see also Breaks: Rest Periods for Expression of Breast Milk (Oregon Bureau of Labor and Industries, Technical Assistance for Employers), http://www.oregon.gov/boli/TA/docs/t_faq_expression_of_breast_milk2.pdf.
[3]Or. Rev. Stat. §§ 659A.150-186.
[4]Or. Rev. Stat. § 653.077
[5]Or. Rev. Stat. § 659A.150(4).
[6]Or. Rev. Stat. § 106.340.

- to care for a newborn or newly adopted child
- to care for a child who is sick (but not seriously ill) and needs care at home[7]

Even if you use the full twelve weeks of leave to care for your new baby, you are still entitled to take as many as twelve *additional weeks* to care for a sick child in the same year.[8]

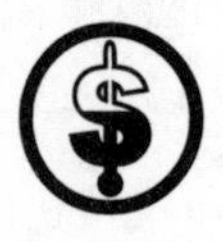

PAID SICK DAYS

The city of Portland requires that all private-sector employees get up to forty hours (five days) of accrued paid sick time (guaranteed time off is unpaid for small businesses with fewer than six employees). Sick time can be used for yourself or to care for a family member, for pregnancy, childbirth, and postpartum care as well as preventive medical care.[9]

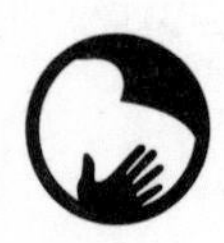

PREGNANCY

Employers with one or more employees may not discriminate in employment on the basis of sex, which includes discrimination because of pregnancy, childbirth, and related medical conditions or occurrences.[10]

If your spouse or partner is pregnant, you also may be protected from employment discrimination based on her pregnancy. That's because the law prohibits employers from discriminating based on the sex, marital status, and sexual orientation (among other characteristics) of any other person with whom you associate.[11]

[7]Or. Rev. Stat. § 659A.159.
[8]Or. Rev. Stat. § 659A.162(2)(b).
[9]Portland Code Tit. 9. Visit www.portlandonline.com for more information.
[10]Or. Rev. Stat. §§ 659A.029, 659A.030. Case law in Oregon also suggests that your employer may not discriminate against you because he or she regards your pregnancy as an impairment. See Melvin v. Kim's Restaurant, Inc., 776 P.2d 1286 (Or. 1989) (finding allegation sufficient to state a claim under disability discrimination law). If your employer has a valid dress code or policy, they may have to make reasonable accommodations for you based on your health and safety needs while you are pregnant. Or. Rev. Stat. § 659A.030(5).
[11]Or. Rev. Stat. § 659A.030(1).

If you work for an employer with twenty-five or more employees, you (as birth mother) may be entitled to twelve weeks of job-protected leave to deal with illness and inability to work related to pregnancy or childbirth. This is in addition to the twelve weeks of leave you may take under the OFLA to care for and bond with a newborn baby.[12]

CAREGIVER DISCRIMINATION

Like the Americans with Disabilities Act, state law in Oregon prohibits an employer from discriminating against a worker because of his or her association with a disabled person.[13] This state law applies to employers with six or more employees.[14]

Eight localities in Oregon (including Portland[15]) prohibit employment discrimination based on familial status or family responsibilities. Check this website to find out whether your city or county provides you with any protections: http://www.worklifelaw.org/pubs/LocalFRDLawsDetail.html.

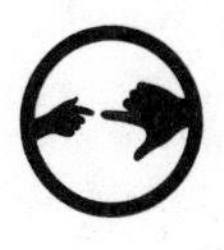

KINCARE

If you are eligible for leave under the Oregon Family Leave Act, you may use your accrued sick leave or other paid leave to care for a new child, a seriously ill family member, or a sick child who requires home care.[16]

See the Paid Sick Days section–accrued sick time may be used for caring for a sick family member.

[12]Or. Rev. Stat. § 659A.162(2)(a).
[13]Or. Rev. Stat. § 659A.112(2)(d).
[14]Or. Rev. Stat. § 659A.106.
[15]Portland, Or. Code § 23.01.050(B).
[16]Or. Rev. Stat. §§ 659A.159, 659A.174.

PUBLIC-SECTOR WORKERS

As a state employee, you may be entitled to even more generous benefits, so be sure to check your employee handbook or union contract or talk with human resources.

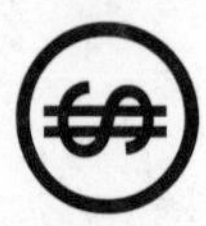

EQUAL PAY

Oregon law prohibits employers from discriminating in pay between men and women doing comparable work.[17]

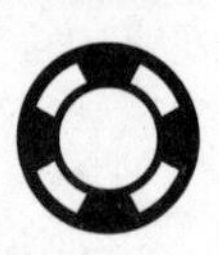

UNEMPLOYMENT INSURANCE

If you lose your job due to the illness or disability of an immediate family member (spouse, domestic partner, parent, or minor child), you may still be eligible for unemployment insurance benefits.[18]

OTHER

Unpaid Bereavement Leave

The Oregon Family Leave Act was amended in 2013 to cover up to two weeks of leave for the death of a family member, including time for a funeral or other service, making arrangements necessitated by the death of the family member, and time for grieving. This leave must be completed within sixty days of receiving notice of the family member's death.[19]

[17]Or. Rev. Stat. § 652.220.
[18]Or. Admin. R. 471-030-0038(1).
[19]Or. Rev. Stat. §§ 659A.156, et. seq.

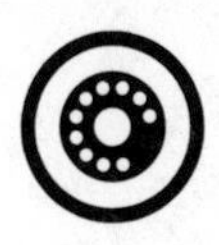

CALL FOR HELP

For questions about discrimination and family leave, and to file a complaint, you can contact the Civil Rights Division of the Oregon Bureau of Labor and Industries:

Phone: 971-673-0764
Address:
800 NE Oregon Street, Suite 1045
Portland, OR 97232
Website: www.oregon.gov/BOLI/CRD/pages/index.aspx
Email: crdemail.boli@state.or.us

Other resources:

Family Forward Oregon
Website: www.familyforwardoregon.org
Email: info@familyforwardoregon.org

PENNSYLVANIA

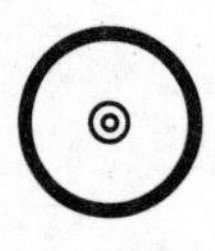

BREASTFEEDING

As a nursing mother, you have the right to breastfeed your child in any private or public place where you and your baby are authorized to be.[1] However, there is no state law expressly protecting your right to express breast milk at work.

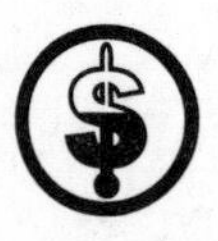

PAID SICK DAYS

If you work for a company that contracts for business with the City of Philadelphia, you may be entitled to a minimum number of paid sick days to recover from your own illness, to access preventive care, or to look after a sick child or family member.[2]

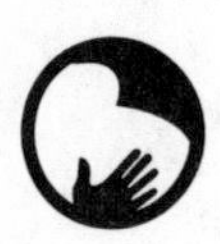

PREGNANCY

State law prohibits employers with four or more employees from discriminating based on sex.[2] The Pennsylvania Human Relations Commission considers discrimination on the basis of maternity or pregnancy to be a form of sex discrimination.[3]

In 2014, Philadelphia passed an ordinance that requires employers to provide reasonable accommodations to employees for needs "related to pregnancy, childbirth, or a related medical condition," so long as such accommodations will not cause an "undue hardship" to the employer.[4] It is the employ-

[1]35 Pa. Stat. § 636.3.
[2]Phila., Pa. Code § 17-305.
[3]43 Pa. Stat. §§ 954, 955.
[4]Pa. Admin. Code § 41.101 to 41.103. The Pennsylvania Human Relations Commission also suggests, in its materials, that you are entitled to a reasonable accommodation of your disability arising from pregnancy or childbirth, unless it poses an undue hardship on your employer. See Having a Baby? Know Your Rights (Pennsylvania Human Relations Commission), http://www.portal.state.pa.us/portal/server.pt/document/933644/pregnancy_discrimination.

er's burden to show that an accommodation would be an undue hardship. The ordinance applies to employers with one or more employees.

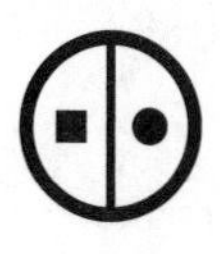

CAREGIVER DISCRIMINATION

Similar to the Americans with Disabilities Act, state law in Pennsylvania prohibits an employer from discriminating against a worker because of his or her relationship with a disabled person.[5] This law applies to employers with four or more employees.

Ten localities in Pennsylvania (including Philadelphia[6]) prohibit employment discrimination based on familial status or family responsibilities.[7]

PUBLIC-SECTOR WORKERS

As a state employee, you may be entitled to even more generous benefits, including unpaid parental leave[8] and family caregiving leave,[9] so be sure to check your employee handbook or union contract or talk with human resources.

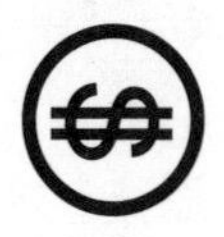

EQUAL PAY

Pennsylvania law forbids employers from discriminating in pay between employees based on sex.[11]

[5]Phila. Code § 9-1128.
[6]43 Pa. Stat. § 955(l).
[7]Phila., Pa. Code § 9-1102.
[8]For more information on local family-friendly laws throughout Pennsylvania, see Terry L. Fromson, et al., *Through the Lens of Equality: Eliminating Sex Bias to Improve the Health of Pennsylvania's Women* (Women's Law Project, 2012), http://www.womenslawproject.org.
[9]Pennsylvania Office of Administration Personnel Rules §§ 8.101-8.112.
[10]Commonwealth of Pennsylvania, Governor's Office, Management Directive 530.30(4)(f), (m) (2007).
[11]43 Pa. Stat. § 336.3.

UNEMPLOYMENT INSURANCE

If you leave your job because of a compelling reason (for example, to care for an ill relative), you may still be eligible for unemployment insurance under Pennsylvania law.[12]

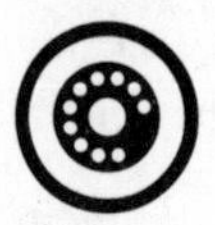

CALL FOR HELP

For questions about discrimination or to file a complaint, you may contact the Pennsylvania Human Relations Commission:

Phone: 717-787-4410
Address:
301 Chestnut Street, Suite 300
Harrisburg, PA 17101-1702
Email: phrc@pa.gov
Website: www.phrc.state.pa.us

Other resources:

Women's Law Project
Phone: 215-928-9801
Address:
125 S. 9th Street, Suite 300
Philadelphia, PA 19107
Email: info@womenslawproject.org
PathWays PA
Phone: 610-543-5022
Website: www.pathwayspa.org

[12] 43 Pa. Stat. § 802; see also McHugh et al., Between a Rock and a Hard Place (July 2003), at http://nelp.3cdn.net/ebba1e75e059fc749d_0um6idptk.pdf.

RHODE ISLAND

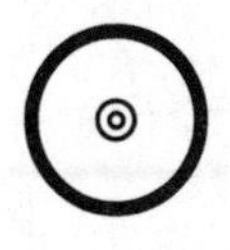

BREASTFEEDING

Rhode Island law allows employers to provide reasonable unpaid break time in an area other than a toilet stall for employees to pump breast milk or breastfeed their babies[1]–but note that this statute is worded in an odd way; it says employers *may* provide this break time but doesn't seem to *require* them to. On the other hand, the private location *shall* be provided. Consult a lawyer about this confusing law.

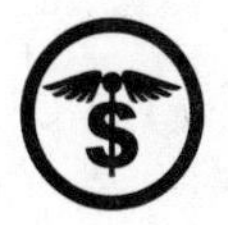

TEMPORARY DISABILITY INSURANCE

Rhode Island is one of just five states to guarantee temporary disability insurance (TDI) for employees, including pregnant women who are unable to work.[2] The program is funded through employee payroll contributions, and benefits may last up to thirty weeks.[3]

While on TDI, you also may be eligible for a "dependents' allowance," which increases your benefit for each of your dependent children under age eighteen.[4] You also may be able to receive partial benefits, if your pregnancy or postpartum disability limits you to part-time work.[5]

[1]R.I. Gen Laws § 23-13.2-1.
[2]R.I. Gen. Laws § 28-41-8.
[3]"Temporary Disability Insurance: Frequently Asked Questions," Rhode Island Department of Labor and Training, accessed January 11, 2013, http://www.dlt.ri.gov/tdi/tdifaqs.htm.
[4]R.I. Gen. Laws § 28-41-5(b).
[5]R.I. Gen. Laws § 28-41-5(d).

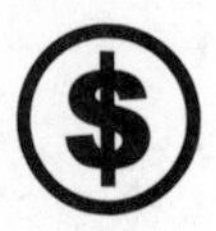

PAID FAMILY LEAVE

Beginning January 1, 2014, Rhode Island's temporary caregiver insurance program (part of the state's temporary disability insurance program) will allow eligible employees to receive partial wage replacement for up to four weeks per year to care for a family member. This benefit can be used to bond with a new child (including foster or adopted children) or to care for a child, spouse, domestic partner, parent, parent-in-law, or grandparent who is seriously ill.

UNPAID FAMILY LEAVE

Some Rhode Island workers are eligible for thirteen weeks of unpaid leave in a two-year period, rather than just the twelve weeks per year under the FMLA, for the birth or adoption of a child, for a family member's serious illness[6] (including a parent, husband, wife, domestic partner, child, or mother- or father-in-law), or to recover from their own serious illness. This additional leave is available if you have worked an average of thirty hours per week for twelve months in a row (1,560 hours), and you work for the State of Rhode Island or any city, town, or municipal agency with thirty or more employees, or if you work for any private employer with fifty or more employees.[7]

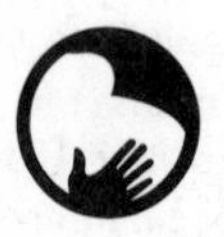

PREGNANCY

If your employer has four or more employees, you are covered by the Rhode Island Fair Employment Practices Act, which outlaws employment discrimination on the basis of sex. This includes discrimination on the basis of pregnancy, childbirth, or related medical conditions.[8] The city of Central Falls passed an ordinance called The Gender Equity in the Workplace Ordinance in April 2014. This new law makes it illegal for an employer to refuse to reasonably accommodate a condition

[6] R.I. Gen. Laws § 28-48-1.
[7] R.I. Gen. Laws §§ 28-48-1(3).
[8] R.I. Gen. Laws § 28-5-6.

related to pregnancy, childbirth, or a related medical condition, among other things.[9]

PARENTAL INVOLVEMENT IN CHILDREN'S EDUCATION

Under the Parental and Family Medical Leave Act, if you have worked an average of thirty hours per week for twelve months in a row (1,560 hours) for a qualifying employer, you can take ten hours every twelve months to attend your child's school conferences or other school-related activities.[9]

This law applies to the State of Rhode Island, to any city, town, or municipal agency with thirty or more employees, and to all private employers with fifty or more employees.[10]

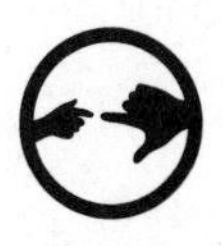

KINCARE

If your employer allows employees to use sick time or sick leave after the birth of their child, you too must be allowed to use sick time in connection with adopting a child under age sixteen.[11]

PUBLIC-SECTOR WORKERS

As a state employee, you may be entitled to more generous benefits, such as use of up to ten paid sick days per year to care for an immediate family member,[12] so be sure to check your employee handbook or union contract or talk with human resources.

[9]Enforcement of this law works differently than others we have discussed. For this law, City Council can revoke or suspend a company's license after three violations. For more information visit http://www.abetterbalance.org/web/images/stories/CF_Protects_Pregnant_Workers_PR_3.pdf.

[10]R.I. Gen. Laws § 28-48-1(3).

[11]R.I. Gen Laws § 28-48-11.

[12]Employee Handbook: Sick Leave with Pay (State of Rhode Island Division of Human Resources, September 22, 2010), http://www.hr.ri.gov/documents/Handbook/leave/1200_Sick%20Leave%20with%20Pay_9-22-2010.pdf.

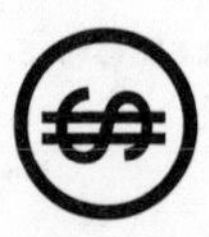

EQUAL PAY

Rhode Island state law specifically prohibits wage discrimination based on sex and applies to nearly all employers, regardless of size.[13]

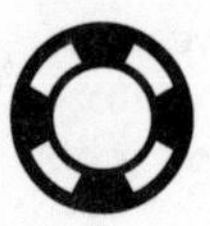

UNEMPLOYMENT INSURANCE

If you lose your job because you need to care for an immediate family member (spouse, parent, parent-in-law, or minor child) who suffers from illness or disability, you may still be eligible for unemployment insurance.[14]

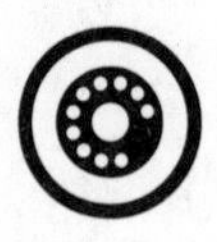

CALL FOR HELP

If you have questions about or think you may be experiencing discrimination at work, you may contact the Rhode Island Commission on Human Rights:

Phone: 401-222-2661
Address:
180 Westminster Street, 3rd Floor
Providence, RI 02903
Website: www.richr.ri.gov

For questions about family and medical leave or temporary disability insurance, contact the Rhode Island Department of Labor and Training:

Website: www.dlt.ri.gov/contact.htm

[13]R.I. Gen. Laws §§ 28-6-17 to 28-6-21.
[14]R.I. Gen. Laws § 28-44-17(a)(3).

SOUTH CAROLINA

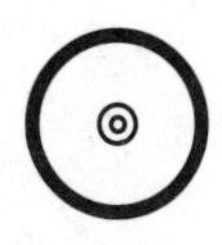

BREASTFEEDING

Although state law allows you to breastfeed your baby in any location where you are authorized to be,[1] there is no law that expressly protects your right to express milk at work.

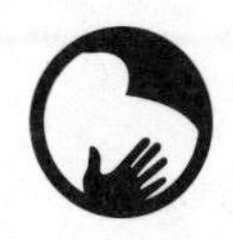

PREGNANCY

The South Carolina Human Affairs Law mirrors Title VII of the Civil Rights Act, banning employers with fifteen or more employees from discriminating in employment based on sex, including pregnancy, childbirth, and related medical conditions.[2]

PUBLIC-SECTOR WORKERS

As a state employee, you may be entitled to more generous benefits, such as use of up to ten paid sick days per year to care for an immediate family member,[3] so be sure to check your employee handbook or union contract or talk with human resources.

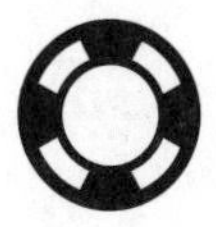

UNEMPLOYMENT INSURANCE

If you leave your job because of the illness or disability of your spouse, parent, or dependent child, you may still be eligible for unemployment insurance benefits.[4]

[1] S.C. Code § 63-5-40.
[2] S.C. Code §§ 1-13-30, 1-30-80.
[3] S.C. Code § 8-11-40.
[4] S.C. Code § 41-35-125(B).

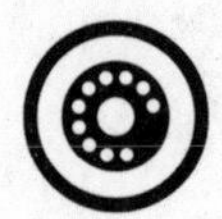

CALL FOR HELP

For questions about discrimination or to file a complaint, you may contact the South Carolina Human Affairs Commission:

Phone: 803-737-7800
Address:
P.O. Box 4490
2611 Forest Drive, Suite 200
Columbia, SC 29204
Email: information@schac.state.sc.us
Website: www.state.sc.us/schac

SOUTH DAKOTA

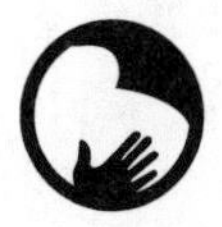

PREGNANCY

South Dakota law bans discrimination on the basis of sex.[1]

The prohibition seems to apply to pregnancy discrimination as well.[2] The law applies to all employers with one employee or more.[3]

PUBLIC-SECTOR WORKERS

As a government employee, you may be entitled to different benefits. Be sure to check your employee handbook or union contract or talk with human resources.

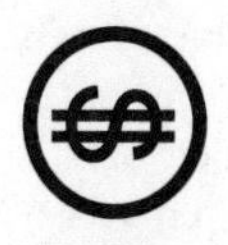

EQUAL PAY

Employers cannot discriminate on the basis of sex in wages.[4]

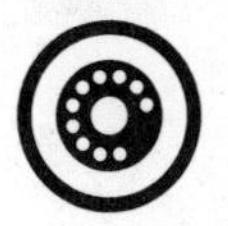

CALL FOR HELP

For questions about the law or to file a complaint, you may contact the South Dakota Division of Human Rights:

Phone: 605-773-3681
Address:
Division of Human Rights (Labor & Management)
South Dakota Department of Labor and Regulation
Kneip Building, 700 Governors Drive
Pierre, SD 57501-2291
Website: dlr.sd.gov/humanrights

[1] S.D. Codified Laws § 20-13-10.
[2] S.D. Admin. R. 20:03:09:12; see also Jones v. American State Bank, 857 F.2d 494, 495 n. 3 (8th Cir. 1988).
[3] S.D. Codified Laws § 20-13-1(7).
[4] S.D. Codified Laws § 60-12-15.

TENNESSEE

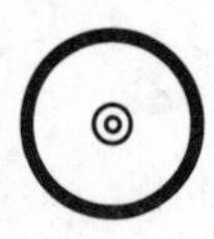

BREASTFEEDING

You can breastfeed your child anywhere you have a right to be.[1]

Employers have to provide reasonable breaks so that you can pump breast milk. They also have to try to find you a private space other than a toilet stall to pump.[2]

UNPAID FAMILY LEAVE

In addition to FMLA rights for workers in businesses of fifty or more employees,[3] employees working for employers with one hundred or more employees who have been with an employer for at least twelve months full-time may take leave for four months for adoption, pregnancy, childbirth, and nursing.[4] You are entitled to the same position, or a similar one, if you give three months' advanced notice, unless it is a medical emergency.[5]

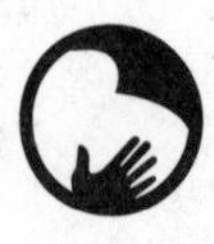

PREGNANCY

Employers with eight or more employees[6] may not discriminate on the basis of sex.[7] The law includes a protection against pregnancy discrimination.[8]

[1]Tenn. Code § 68-58-101.
[2]Tenn. Code § 50-1-305.
[3]Tenn. Code § 4-21-408(d)(2).
[4]Tenn. Code § 4-21-408(a).
[5]Tenn. Code § 4-21-408(b)(2). If you unexpectedly got notice of adoption, then you also might not be required to provide three months' notice. Tenn. Code § 4-21-408(b)(3).
[6]Tenn. Code § 4-21-102(5).
[7]Tenn. Code § 4-21-401.
[8]Tenn. Code § 4-21-101(a)(1); see also Spann v. Abraham, 36 S.W.3d 452, 462 (Tenn. Ct. App. 1999).

PUBLIC-SECTOR WORKERS

As a government employee, you may be entitled to more generous benefits, such as taking off up to one day per month to participate in your child's school,[9] so be sure to check your employee handbook or union contract or talk with human resources.

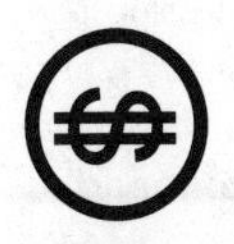

EQUAL PAY

Employers cannot discriminate between employees in wages in the same establishment on the basis of sex alone.[10]

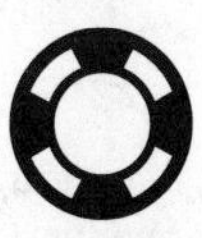

UNEMPLOYMENT INSURANCE

If you have to leave work because of pregnancy, then you might still qualify for benefits with medical documentation.[11]

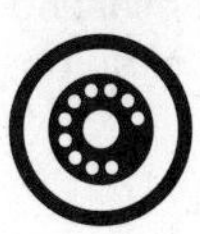

CALL FOR HELP

For more information about your rights, or to file a complaint, you may contact the Tennessee Human Rights Commission:

> **Phone:** 615-741-5825
> **Address:**
> 710 James Robertson Parkway, Suite 100
> Corner of Rosa Parks Blvd.
> Nashville, TN 37243-1219
> **Website:** www.tn.gov/humanrights

If you work in Tennessee, you can also contact our A Better Balance Southern Office, at 615-915-2417, regarding any questions about your workplace rights as an expecting or new parent.

[9]Tenn. Code § 49-6-7001.
[10]Tenn. Code § 50-2-202.
[11]Tenn. Code § 50-7-303(a)(1)(A).

TEXAS

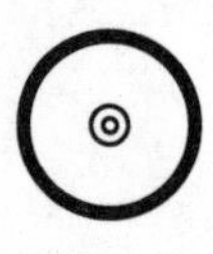

BREASTFEEDING

Although state law protects your right to breastfeed your baby in any location you are authorized to be,[1] there is no state law that specifically protects your right to express milk at work. However, businesses that implement policies supporting workplace breastfeeding may use the term "mother-friendly" in their promotional materials.[2]

PREGNANCY

Texas law mirrors Title VII of the Civil Rights Act, banning employers with fifteen or more employees from discriminating in employment based on sex, including pregnancy, childbirth, and related medical conditions.[3]

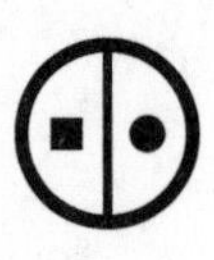

CAREGIVER DISCRIMINATION

The city of Chico may not discriminate in employment based on familial status, which includes pregnancy, parental/guardian status, and adoption of a child.[4] This law applies only to the city and its employees and officers.

PUBLIC-SECTOR WORKERS

As a state employee, you may be entitled to more generous benefits, such as parental leave,[5] time off to attend parent-teacher conferences,[6] and use of paid sick time to care for an immediate family member,[7] so be sure to check your employee handbook or union contract or talk with human resources.

[1]Tex. Health & Safety Code § 165.002.
[2]Tex. Health & Safety Code § 165.003.
[3]Tex. Lab. Code §§ 21.002(8), 21.051, 21.106.
[4]Chico, Tex. Code § 31.40-.41.
[5]Tex. Gov't. Code § 661.913.
[6]Tex. Gov't. Code § 661.206.
[7]Tex. Gov't. Code § 661.202(d).

If you work for municipal or county government, and your doctor recommends certain restrictions for your work during pregnancy, you may be entitled to a workplace accommodation, including an alternative, temporary work assignment.[8]

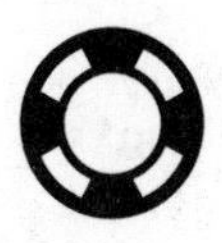

UNEMPLOYMENT INSURANCE

If you lose your job because of the illness of a minor child or terminal illness of a spouse, or because of your own pregnancy, you may still be eligible for unemployment insurance.[9]

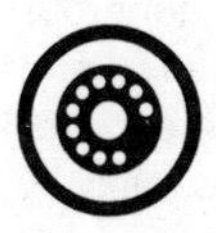

OTHER

Texas has a state Work and Family Clearinghouse that provides information and links to resources on work-family programs and policies for employers, employees, policy makers, and the public. You can access the information through the Texas Workforce Commission at its website: http://www.twc.state.tx.us/svcs/workfamch/wfchp.html.

CALL FOR HELP

For questions about employment discrimination, or to file a complaint, you may contact the Civil Rights Division of the Texas Workforce Commission:

Phone: 512-463-2642
Website: www.twc.state.tx.us

[8]Tex. Loc. Gov't. Code § 180.004.
[9]Tex. Lab. Code §§ 207.046(a)(3), 207.045(d)(1) & (4), 207.045(e).

UTAH

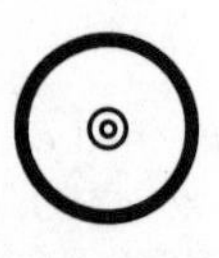

BREASTFEEDING

Although your right to breastfeed in public is generally protected under state law,[1] there is no specific law protecting your right to express breast milk at work.

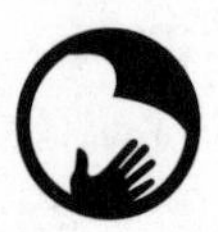

PREGNANCY

The Utah Antidiscrimination Act tracks Title VII of the Civil Rights Act of 1964, making it illegal for an employer with fifteen or more employees to discriminate against someone on the basis of sex, pregnancy, childbirth, and pregnancy-related conditions.[2]

PUBLIC-SECTOR WORKERS

As a state employee, you may be entitled to more generous benefits, such as use of sick time for preventive health and dental care, for maternity/paternity and adoption care, or for absence because of illness, injury, or temporary disability of a spouse or dependents living in your home,[3] so be sure to check your employee handbook or union contract or talk with human resources.

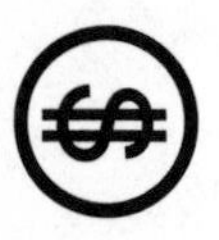

EQUAL PAY

The Utah Antidiscrimination Act prohibits payment of different wages to employees who have substantially equal experience, responsibilities, and skill, because of their sex or because of pregnancy, childbirth, or pregnancy-related conditions.[4]

[1]Utah Code Ann. §§ 17-15-25, § 76-10-1229.5.
[2]Utah Code Ann. §§ 34A-5-102, 34A-5-106.
[3]Utah Admin. Code R477-7-4.
[4]Utah Code Ann. § 34A-5-106(1)(a)(iii)(A).

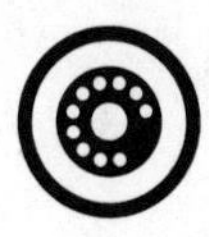

CALL FOR HELP

For questions about employment discrimination, or to file a complaint, you may contact the Utah Labor Commission, Anti-discrimination and Labor Division:

Phone: 801-530-6801
Address:
160 East 300 South, 3rd Floor
Salt Lake City, UT 84111
Email: discrimination@utah.gov
Website: laborcommission.utah.gov

VERMONT

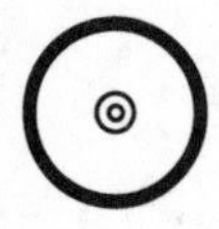

BREASTFEEDING

In addition to guaranteeing your right to breastfeed your child in any place of public accommodation where you and your child otherwise have the right to be,[1] Vermont requires all employers to provide reasonable time throughout the day for nursing mothers to express breast milk for three years after giving birth. Employers must also make reasonable accommodations to provide appropriate private space (not a bathroom stall) where nursing moms can pump and may not discriminate against employees who exercise their rights under the law.[2]

UNPAID FAMILY LEAVE

The "parental leave" part of Vermont's Parental and Family Leave Act (PFLA) covers employers with ten or more workers and provides up to twelve weeks of leave during your pregnancy and/or after childbirth, or within a year after you adopt a child sixteen years or younger.[3]

The "family leave" part of the PFLA covers employers with fifteen or more workers and provides up to twelve weeks of leave to recover from your own serious illness or to care for your seriously ill child, civil union partner, parent, spouse (including same-sex spouse), or parent-in-law.[4]

[1]Vt. Stat. tit. 9, § 4502(j).
[2]Vt. Stat. tit. 21, § 305. "An Act Relating to Equal Pay" (H.99) strengthens the anti-retaliation provision in 21 V.S.A. § 305.
[3]Vt. Stat. tit. 21, §§ 471-472.
[4]Vt. Stat. tit. 21, §§ 471-472; tit. 15, § 1204.

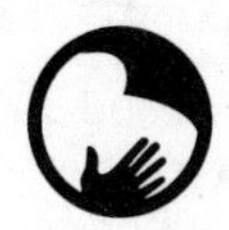

PREGNANCY

The Vermont Fair Employment Practices Act makes it illegal for employers with one or more workers to discriminate in employment on the basis of sex.[5] Although the statute does not specifically prohibit discrimination based on pregnancy, the Supreme Court of Vermont has interpreted the law that way.[6]

PARENTAL INVOLVEMENT IN CHILDREN'S EDUCATION

If you work for an employer with fifteen or more workers, the "Short-Term Family Leave" section of the PFLA may entitle you to up to four hours in any thirty-day period (but not more than twenty-four hours in any twelve-month period) of short-term, unpaid leave to participate in preschool or school activities directly related to the academic advancement of your child, stepchild, foster child, or ward who lives with you.[7]

KINCARE

If you work for an employer with fifteen or more workers, you also may use some of the time guaranteed by the Short-Term Family Leave section of the PFLA to:

- attend or accompany your child, stepchild, foster child, or ward who lives with you or your parent, spouse, or parent-in-law to routine medical or dental appointments;
- accompany your parent, spouse, or parent-in-law to other appointments for professional services related to their care and well-being; or
- respond to a medical emergency involving your child, stepchild, foster child, or ward who lives with you or your parent, spouse, or parent-in-law.

[5]Vt. Stat. tit. 21, § 495.
[6]Woolaver v. State, 833 A.2d 849, 860 (Vt. 2003) ("We have held that pregnancy discrimination qualifies as sex discrimination under FEPA ..." [citing Lavalley v. E.B. & A.C. Whiting Co., 692 A.2d 367, 370-31 (Vt. 1997)]).
[7]Vt. Stat. tit. 21, § 472A.

PUBLIC-SECTOR WORKERS

As a state employee, you may be entitled to more generous benefits, such as four months of unpaid leave following the birth of a child and use of accrued sick leave for any period of disability prior to childbirth and for up to six weeks after childbirth,[8] so be sure to check your employee handbook or union contract or talk with human resources.

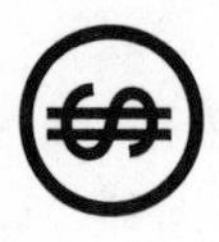

EQUAL PAY

Vermont law prohibits employers from discriminating between employees on the basis of sex by paying wages to employees of one sex at a rate less than the rate paid to employees of the other sex for equal work that requires equal skill, effort, and responsibility and that is performed under similar working conditions.[9]

Your employer may not discriminate against you for disclosing the amount of your wages and cannot require, as a condition of employment, that you not disclose the amount you earn.[10]

Employers seeking to justify a sex-based pay differential by asserting a bona fide factor other than sex must demonstrate that the factor does not perpetuate a sex-based differential in compensation, is job-related with respect to the position in question, and is based upon a legitimate business consideration.

Employers cannot prevent employees from disclosing their wages or from inquiring about or discussing the wages of other employees.

OTHER

Flexible Work Arrangements

An employee may request a flexible working arrangement that meets the needs of the employer and employee. The employer shall consider such a request using the given procedures at least twice per calendar year (Effective January 1, 2014)[11]

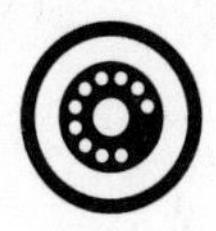

CALL FOR HELP

If you work for a private employer and have concerns about workplace discrimination, or if you want more information about the Vermont Parental and Family Leave Act, contact the Vermont Attorney General Civil Rights Unit:

Phone: 888-745-9195
Website: www.atg.state.vt.us

If you work for the state and suspect discrimination, you may contact the Vermont Human Rights Commission:

Phone: 800-416-2010, ext. 25
Address:
14-16 Baldwin Street
Montpelier, VT 05633-6301
Email: human.rights@state.vt.us
Website: http://hrc.vermont.gov

VIRGINIA

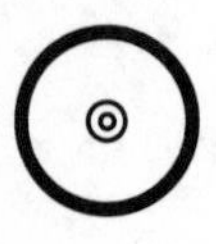

BREASTFEEDING

You have the right to breastfeed your child on any property where you are allowed to be that is owned, leased, or controlled by the state.[1]

An employer cannot fire[2] you because of a childbirth-related condition, including lactation, defined to mean both feeding a child directly and expressing milk.[3] This law applies to employers with more than five but fewer than fifteen employees.[4]

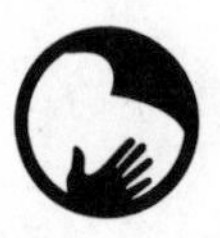

PREGNANCY

Virginia prohibits employers with more than five but fewer than fifteen employees from firing[5] an employee because of sex, pregnancy, childbirth, or related medical conditions.[6]

The law also specifically mentions that "sex or gender" includes pregnancy, childbirth, and related medical conditions. It goes on to state that pregnant women and women giving birth must be treated the same as others similar in their abilities.[7]

[1]Va. Code § 2.2-1147.1.
[2]It is unusual that the statute mentions only firing ("discharge") and no other forms of discrimination, such as demotions. At least one court has said that this means the law prohibits only firing. See Porter v. Elk Remodeling, Inc., No. 1:09-cv-446, 2010 WL 2346625 at *8 (E.D.Va. June 9, 2010).
[3]Va. Code § 2.2-3903.
[4]Ibid.
[5]See footnote 2 of this section about the fact that the statute only mentions firing.
[6]Va. Code § 2.2-3903.
[7]Va. Code § 2.2-3901.

PUBLIC-SECTOR WORKERS

As a state employee, you may be entitled to more generous benefits, such as short-term disability benefits for some employees during maternity leave,[8] so be sure to check your employee handbook or union contract or talk with human resources.

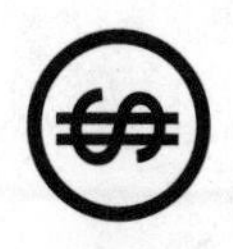

EQUAL PAY

Employers in Virginia may not discriminate against employees on the basis of sex by paying lower wages.[9]

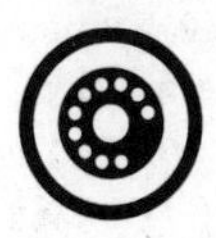

CALL FOR HELP

For questions about the law or to file a complaint, you may contact the Virginia Division of Human Rights:

Phone: 804-225-2292
Address:
Division of Human Rights
Office of the Attorney General
900 East Main Street
Richmond, VA 23219
Email: human_rights@oag.state.va.us
Website: www.oag.state.va.us/Programs%20and%20 Resources/Human_Rights

[8] Va. Code § 51.1-1110.
[9] Va. Code § 40.1-28.6.

WASHINGTON

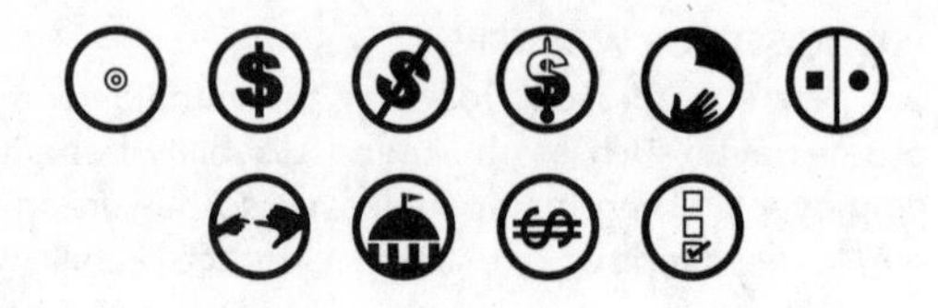

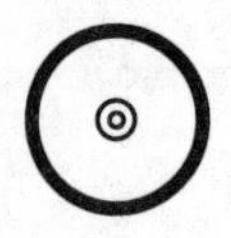

BREASTFEEDING

You have the right to be free from discrimination[1] while breastfeeding your child in any public place.[2]

Employers who have a workplace breastfeeding policy that has been approved by the department of health may use the designation of "infant-friendly" on their promotional materials.[3]

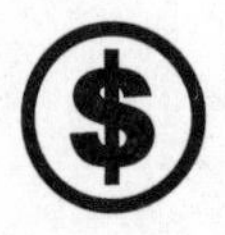

PAID FAMILY LEAVE

Washington passed a family leave insurance program to provide up to five weeks per year of wage replacement for workers to use while caring for a newborn child or a newly placed adopted child.[4] The law will not be implemented until October 2015.

Once the law goes into effect, you will be eligible for family leave insurance if you have been employed for at least 680 hours during your qualifying year.[5] The benefit amount will start at $250/week for any individual working at least thirty-five hours per week, with a prorated payment schedule for those employees working fewer than thirty-five hours per week.[6]

[1]Wash. Rev. Code § 49.60.215.
[2]Wash. Rev. Code § 49.60.030(g).
[3]Wash. Rev. Code § 43.70.640.
[4]Wash. Rev. Code. § 49.86.005–49.86.903.
[5]Wash. Rev. Code § 49.86.030.
[6]Wash. Rev. Code § 49.86.060.

UNPAID FAMILY LEAVE

The Washington State Family Leave Act (FLA) covers the same ground as the FMLA and expands on it in three ways:

- If you take leave from work for pregnancy-related conditions or childbirth and qualify for leave under the federal FMLA, you are entitled to additional leave benefits under the FLA. Qualified employees will receive twelve weeks of state family leave in addition to the pregnancy disability leave ordered by their health care providers.[7]
- The law covers care for an employee's state-registered domestic partner and for the child of an employee's domestic partner.[8] Same-sex spouses are also covered.
- If you take FMLA for a qualifying exigency related to a military deployment or as a military caregiver, then you could qualify for all twelve weeks of leave under FLA.[9]

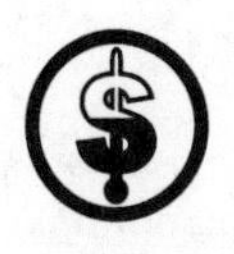

PAID SICK DAYS

Certain employees in Seattle are now entitled to accrue paid sick time. The amount of time workers can take off depends on the size of the employer.[10]

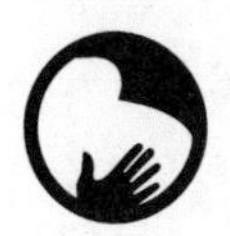

PREGNANCY

It is an unfair employment practice for an employer (public or private with eight or more employees) to refuse to hire or promote a woman, to terminate or demote a woman, or to impose different terms and conditions of employment on a woman because of pregnancy or childbirth unless the employer can demonstrate a business necessity for doing so.[11] An employer also may not discriminate against a woman based on her potential to become pregnant.[12]

[7]Wash. Rev. Code § 49.78.390; Washington State Family Leave Act Q&A (Washington State Department of Labor and Industries, March 2010), http://www.lni.wa.gov/WorkplaceRights/files/FamilyLeaveFAQs.pdf.

[8]Wash. Rev. Code § 49.78.020(1), (7), & 17; § 49.78.904.

[9]Washington State Family Leave Act Q&A, 2.

[10]Seattle, Wash. Code § 14.16.01 et seq.

[11]Wash. Rev. Code § 49.60.180; Wash. Admin. Code § 162-30-020(3).

[12]Wash. Admin. Code § 162-30-020(2)(a).

It is also illegal to base employment decisions or actions on negative assumptions about pregnant women.[13]

If your employer has eight or more employees, it must also provide a leave of absence for the time you are sick or disabled because of pregnancy or childbirth and must return you to the same or similar job with at least the same pay.[14]

CAREGIVER DISCRIMINATION
In Tacoma, Washington, it is unlawful for an employer to require an applicant to provide information regarding familial status.[15]

KINCARE
Employers are required to allow employees to use sick time or other paid leave to care for a sick child, spouse, parent, parent-in-law, or grandparent.[16]

PUBLIC-SECTOR WORKERS
As a government employee, you may be entitled to more generous benefits, so be sure to check your employee handbook or union contract or talk with human resources.

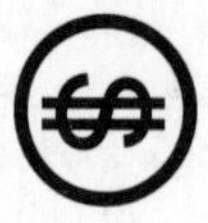

EQUAL PAY
Employers cannot discriminate between the sexes in wage payments.[17]

[13] Wash. Admin. Code § 162-30-020(3)(c).
[14] Wash. Admin. Code § 162-30-020(4); See Hegwine v. Longview Fibre Co., 172 P.3d 688, 693 (Wash. 2007) (noting that the Washington Human Rights Commission's regulations, interpreting and enforcing the Washington Law against Discrimination, deserve "great weight" in judicial decisions); see also Johnson v. Goodyear Tire & Rubber Co., 790 F. Supp. 1516 (E.D. Wash. 1992) (construing WAC 162-30-020 liberally to accomplish the purposes for which it was adopted—namely, "to spare a woman the dilemma of choosing between work and family" and finding that defendant violated the regulation by assigning plaintiff to a less secure job upon return from her maternity leave).
[15] Tacoma, Wash. Code § 1.29.050(A).
[16] Wash. Rev. Code § 49.12.270.
[17] Wash. Rev. Code § 49.12.175.

OTHER

Washington law says that employers must grant adoptive parents and stepparents (both men and women) the same amount of leave time that they provide for biological parents (not counting maternity disability leave).[18]

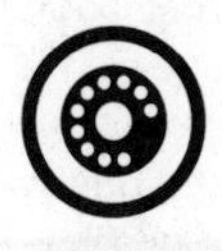

CALL FOR HELP

For questions about the law or to file a complaint, you may contact the Washington State Human Rights Commission:

Phone: 360-753-6770 / TDD: 800-300-7525
Address:
711 S. Capitol Way, Suite 402
Olympia, WA 98504-2490
Website: http://www.hum.wa.gov

[18] Wash. Rev. Code § 49.12.360.

WEST VIRGINIA

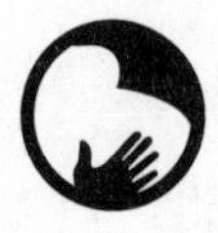

PREGNANCY

The West Virginia Human Rights Act prohibits discrimination on the basis of sex,[1] which seems to include pregnancy.[2] The law applies to those employers with twelve or more employees.[3] The West Virginia Pregnant Workers Fairness Act requires employers to provide reasonable accommodations to employees for limitations related to pregnancy, childbirth, or related medical conditions.[4]

PUBLIC-SECTOR WORKERS

As a government employee, you may be entitled to more generous benefits, such as those provided by the Parental Leave Act,[5] so be sure to check your employee handbook or union contract or talk with human resources.

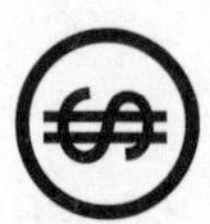

EQUAL PAY

Employers can't discriminate in terms of wages on the basis of sex.[6]

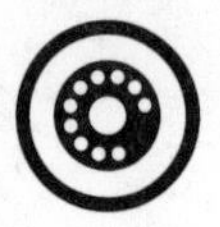

CALL FOR HELP

For questions about the law or to file a complaint you may contact the West Virginia Human Rights Commission:

Phone: 304-558-2616
Address:
1321 Plaza East, Room 108A
Charleston, WV 25301-1400
Website: http://www.hrc.wv.gov

[1] W. Va. Code §§ 5-11-9; 5-11-3(h).
[2] See, for example, Frank's Shoe Store v. West Virginia Human Rights Com'n, 365 S.E.2d 251 (W. Va. 1986).
[3] W. Va. Code § 5-11-3(d).
[4] 2014 WV HB 4284.
[5] W. Va. Code § 21-5D-4.
[6] W. Va. Code § 21-5B-3.

WISCONSIN

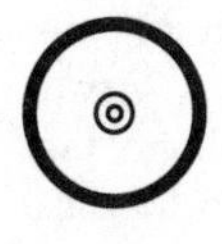

BREASTFEEDING

A mother has the right to breastfeed her child anywhere she is authorized to be; no one can restrict a mother from breastfeeding.[1]

UNPAID FAMILY LEAVE

Private-sector workers have slightly greater access to family and medical leave under Wisconsin law than under the federal FMLA. The Wisconsin law applies to workers who have worked for an employer of fifty or more employees[2] for at least one thousand hours over the preceding year[3] and defines family more broadly than the federal FMLA to include domestic partners. However, state law provides less generous amounts of time off than the federal FMLA. Workers are entitled to a maximum of six weeks of leave to care for a new child, up to two weeks of leave to care for a spouse or domestic partner with a serious health condition, and up to two weeks of pregnancy-related leave in any twelve-month period.[4]

You can also take two weeks off for your own serious health condition, if you aren't able to work.[5] "Serious health condition" is defined to include a disabling condition involving inpatient care in a hospital or outpatient care requiring continuing supervision by a health care provider,[6] so pregnancy and childbirth may qualify.

[1]Wis. Stat. § 253.165.
[2]Wis. Stat. § 103.10(1)(c).
[3]Wis. Stat. § 103.10(2)(c).
[4]Wis. Stat. § 103.10(3).
[5]Wis. Stat. § 103.10(4).
[6]Wis. Stat. § 103.10(1)(g).

Employees can substitute any accrued leave for unpaid family or medical leave.[7]

Like the FMLA, this law has many provisions and some of the details are more favorable than the FMLA. If you would like to take advantage of this law, then you will have to do your homework to really understand the details. The Wisconsin Department of Workforce Development maintains a website that compares the benefits of the Wisconsin Family and Medical Leave Act and the FMLA, which is useful in determining what your coverage would be under both laws.

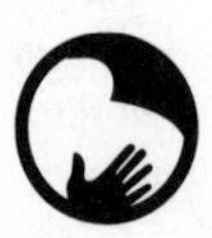

PREGNANCY

The law bans discrimination on the basis of sex,[8] and "sex" is defined to include pregnancy, childbirth, and maternity leave.[9] It applies to employers with at least one employee.[10]

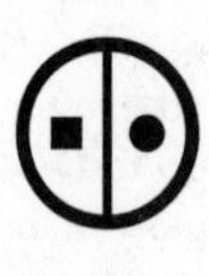

CAREGIVER DISCRIMINATION

Milwaukee and Racine might prohibit discrimination on the basis of familial status,[11] but we were unable to verify that this is the case. Check with a local lawyer to find out more.

PUBLIC-SECTOR WORKERS

As a government employee, you may be entitled to more generous benefits, so be sure to check your employee handbook or union contract or talk with human resources.

[7]Wis. Stat. § 103.10(5)(b).
[8]Wis. Stat. §§ 111.321; 111.322.
[9]Wis. Stat. § 111.36(1)(c).
[10]Wis. Stat. § 111.32(6).
[11]See Stephanie Bornstein & Robert J. Rathmell, Caregivers as a Protected Class?: The Growth of State and Local Laws Prohibiting Family Responsibilities Discrimination (The Center for Worklife Law, December 2009), http://www.worklifelaw.org/pubs/LocalFRDLawsDetail.html.

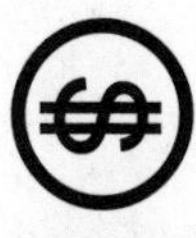

EQUAL PAY

Discriminating on the basis of sex in compensation for equal or substantially similar work is illegal.[12]

UNEMPLOYMENT INSURANCE

You might still be eligible for benefits if you had to leave work because of a verified illness or disability of an immediate family member.[13]

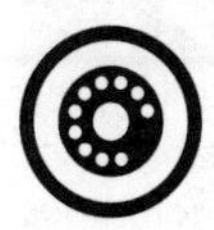

CALL FOR HELP

For more information about the law or to file a complaint, you may contact the Wisconsin Equal Rights Division:

Phone: 608-266-6860 / TTY: 608-264-8752
Address:
201 E. Washington Avenue, Room A300
P.O. Box 8928
Madison, WI 53708
Website: dwd.wisconsin.gov/er/equal_rights_division

Other resources:

9to5, National Association of Working Women
Phone: 414-274-0925
Address:
207 E. Buffalo, Suite 211
Milwaukee WI 53202
Email: 9to5Milwaukee@9to5.org
Website: www.9to5.org/local/milwaukee

[12]Wis. Stat. § 111.36(1)(a).
[13]Wis. Stat. § 108.04.

WYOMING

PREGNANCY

Wyoming law specifically prohibits discrimination on the basis of pregnancy[1] for all employers with two or more employees (unless the employer is a religious organization).[2]

Additionally, while there are no specific laws or regulations on the issue of pregnancy accommodations under state law, the Department of Workforce Services' Labor Standards has chosen to rely on EEOC guidelines which require accommodations for women facing temporary "complications from pregnancy" that fall within the definition of a "disability."[3]

PUBLIC-SECTOR WORKERS

As a government employee, you may be entitled to more generous benefits, so be sure to check your employee handbook or union contract or talk with human resources.

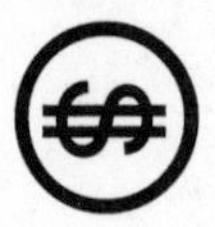

EQUAL PAY

Men and women must be paid the same for equal work.[4]

[1]Wyo. Stat. § 27-9-105(a).
[2]Wyo. Stat. § 27-9-102(b).
[3]Email from Cherie Doak, deputy administrator of the Wyoming Department of Workforce Services' Labor Standards Office, to Liz Reiner Platt (Dec. 10, 2013, 12:07 EST) (on file with author).
[4]Wyo. Stat. § 27-4-302.[1]Wyo. Stat. § 27-9-105(a).

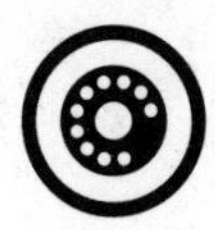

CALL FOR HELP

For questions about the law the Wyoming Department of Workforce Services' Labor Standards Office:

Phone: 307-777-7261
Address:
Labor Standards (Main Office)
1510 East Pershing Boulevard, West Wing, #150
Cheyenne, WY 82002
Website: www.wyomingworkforce.org

ACKNOWLEDGMENTS

We are grateful to all the people who helped make this book possible and who encouraged us along the way.

Thank you to our colleagues Sherry Leiwant, Jared Make, and Risha Foulkes for their insight and encouragement as we drafted and redrafted these chapters. *Babygate* represents their work too, as skillful and dedicated advocates for working families. Special thanks to Liz Reiner Platt and Rachel Sica, who helped shape this book into its current form.

Thank you as well to A Better Balance's board of directors, which has championed our efforts in countless ways over the past nine years, in particular cofounders and board stalwarts Yolanda Wu, Risa Kaufman, and Roslyn Powell. We are also thankful for our advisory board, with special gratitude to Ann Crittenden and Joan Williams, who inspired A Better Balance's founders to launch this organization in 2005.

We are supremely grateful for the generosity of our volunteers—Chelsea Levinson, Melissa Paquette, Jennie Rothman, and Joo Young Seo—who tirelessly researched state and federal law and reviewed our drafts, providing thoughtful feedback and suggestions. Marcella Kocolatos also contributed invaluable research to our state-by-state guide. And we thank J. J. Rudisill and Suki Boynton for their illustrations, which added so much to *Babygate*. We also are indebted to Cynthia Calvert for reviewing our manuscript in its final stages and offering suggestions for improvements based on her wealth of experience.

Thank you to our partners at Outten & Golden LLP, who work with us to provide free consultations to low-income New Yorkers about problems at work related to their family responsibilities. We have learned from and become more effective advocates thanks to their expertise, and their support has allowed us to expand our capacity to help even more workers in need of legal advice.

Babygate would not have been the same without the families we have met through our advocacy. Their stories inspired us to launch this project and offer powerful testimony throughout our book. Although we won't thank them by name, we offer our sincerest gratitude to all the individuals who shared their experiences with us and whose courage in the face of discrimination inspires us each day.

Our work at A Better Balance would not have been possible without the generosity of our funders, including the hundreds of individuals who support us each year. We particularly want to thank the Ford Foundation, which has funded A Better Balance since our infancy as an organization and which continues to sustain our work.

Finally, we want to thank our own families for their love, patience, and guidance as we embarked on our maiden book-writing voyage. As mothers, daughters, and wives, we live the challenges of work–family balance as much as we work to solve them, and we are eternally grateful to our families for supporting us in both endeavors.

DISCUSSION QUESTIONS

Creating Community around *Babygate*

Are you a member of a book club? A mom's group? Read *Babygate* with your friends and start a conversation about maternity leave, flexible work, pregnancy discrimination, and how, together, we can change the way America works.

1. Why do you think the United States is such an outlier in the world regarding public policies to support the unpaid labor of working parents? How does this make you feel as a citizen/taxpayer/parent? How can we, as individuals, change this culture?
2. What do you find to be the most challenging aspects of navigating the workplace as a pregnant or new parent? If you are not yet pregnant or a parent, what worries you most as you think about taking that step? Have you felt the work–family crunch in other ways unrelated to parenting?
3. What solutions or strategies have you successfully employed to help you manage the demands of work and home? What resources do you wish you had to help you in that effort?
4. After reviewing the state-by-state guide, does anything surprise you? What opportunities to you see for improvement?

5. What do you think are the best arguments for convincing employers, businesses, and policy makers to invest in working parents and their families?
6. What action items do you feel that you, or your fellow group members, might be able to take to help change the culture of American workplaces and/or the laws in our country so that they value families?

We hope these questions spark a lively discussion and we're eager to hear what you come up with in your brainstorming. Please email us your ideas and comments at babygate@abetterbalance.org and join the conversation!